THE PSORIASIS CURE

LISA LeVAN

AVERY PUBLISHING GROUP

Garden City Park • New York

The information, advice, and procedures contained in this book are based upon the research and the personal and professional experiences of the author. They are not intended as a substitute for consulting with your physician or other health-care provider. The publisher and author are not responsible for any adverse effects or consequences resulting from the use of any of the suggestions, preparations, or procedures discussed in this book. All matters pertaining to your physical health should be supervised by a health-care professional. It is a sign of wisdom, not cowardice, to seek a second or third opinion.

Cover designer: Doug Brooks
In-house editor: Dara Stewart
Typesetter: Richard Morrock
Printer: Paragon Press, Honesdale, PA

Avery Publishing Group
120 Old Broadway
Garden City Park, NY 11040
1–800–548–5757
www.averypublishing.com

Library of Congress Cataloging-in-Publication Data

LeVan, Lisa.
    The psoriasis cure: a drug-free guide to stopping and reversing the symptoms of psoriasis/ Lisa LeVan.
        p. cm
    Includes bibliographical references and index.
    ISBN 0-89529-917-8
    1. Psoriasis—Treatment Popular works. 2. Psoriasis—Prevention Popular works. I. Title.
    RL321.L48 1999
    616.5′26—dc21

                                                                99-28980
                                                                CIP

Printed in the United States of America

10   9   8   7   6   5   4   3   2   1

Contents

This book is dedicated to my father (from whom I got my psoriasis) and mother, who have always supported me in all my endeavors, and my son. This book was written to help my beloved son, who is likely to have psoriasis when he gets older, and others around the world who already suffer from psoriasis.

Introduction

Psoriasis is more than just a skin disorder. Sufferers often feel disfigured, and shy away from others. Embarrassment leads to emotional stress, and this worsens the condition. Psoriasis is a reflection of conditions that affect much more than the skin.

Up until now, doctors in the United States thought that psoriasis was incurable. That's why commonly prescribed treatments are strictly focused on symptoms. These treatments are designed only to relieve symptoms and prevent secondary infections, without addressing the true causes of the condition or the things going on in the body.

Control of psoriasis requires treating more than just the skin. Traditional medicine has tunnel vision, centered on creams, lotions, and steroids. Many of these traditional treatments are more than just questionable—they are downright dangerous! Each year, thousands of people die from adverse effects of steroids and light therapy. Using physician-prescribed treatments can be your written death sentence.

Psoriasis is not just skin deep. This fact makes standard medical treatment very limited because standard medical treatment focuses on the skin, treats only the symptoms of psoriasis, and typically causes undesired side effects.

There is hope for you, however. Through my research of scientific literature, I have found several natural nutritional supplements that many psoriasis sufferers respond well to. There is considerable evidence that diet plays a critical role in the health of your body and your skin. Eating the right things will decrease, and then slowly eliminate, the inflammation. Eating the wrong things and not taking in the things your body is screaming for increases the inflammation.

I have developed and used the program described in this book on myself and others, and have seen impressive results. Some of these people had been unable to get relief from, or could not tolerate, traditional psoriasis treatments. Some now enjoy life symptom-free.

This book is designed to give you answers. The first chapter explains what psoriasis is, how your body's ability to handle fat affects psoriasis, the symptoms of psoriasis and which parts of your body are affected, what causes psoriasis, how you can tell if you have psoriasis, and how it is different from other skin problems. Chapter 2 explains why you get psoriasis and what is really happening inside your body when you see flakes on your skin. Chapter 3 explains how traditional treatments can hurt you more than they help you. Chapter 4 gives you new hope for beating your psoriasis by explaining what works and how it works. Chapters 5, 6, 7, and 8 give you simple, easy-to-use guidelines for living a life free from psoriasis. This information examines very safe methods based on published scientific and medical research.

There are some points that you should keep in mind if you choose to follow the Psoriasis Cure program:

- Psoriasis is a truly variable condition; every person is unique and responds differently to treatment, so it is possible that what works for many may not work for you.

- If you have had severe psoriasis for years, you will not get rid of all your symptoms overnight. You didn't get all of your symptoms overnight, and it will take time to slowly heal your damaged body. However, the program described in this book may still offer you dramatic relief. This program is a safer and perhaps more effective treatment alternative than most standard physician-prescribed therapies.

- There are several medical conditions that mimic some of the symptoms of psoriasis. In addition, psoriasis is often a symptom of an underlying disorder. When you treat the underlying medical condition, your symptoms may disappear forever. For these reasons, a thorough and accurate examination and diagnosis are critical to determine the best treatment.

You no longer have to put up with the physical and emotional discomfort of psoriasis. Read on to discover safe and natural ways to start getting rid of your symptoms and to start healing the problems in your body that cause your psoriasis.

1

What Is Psoriasis?

It starts with a little redness on your elbows, face, or knees. No big deal. Then, you notice it feels dry and is starting to flake. You even sometimes find yourself rubbing or scratching the spot. You've got your first date since starting college this Friday night, and that mess on your face and elbows has got to go!

You try putting some moisturizer on the spot and rubbing off the scales, but in the morning, the scales are back, and the spot is redder and bigger. Everything you try just seems to make it more noticeable. Just when you think things can't get worse, you notice *another* red spot. You're becoming desperate—desperate enough to call home and ask mom and dad for help.

"Dad! I've got this horrible-looking flaky red spot on my face, and I can't make it go away. I've tried everything. Any ideas?"

"Have you eaten any bacon lately?"

"Well, yeah. The school serves breakfast every morning in the cafeteria, and I've been having some every morning. It's really good. I wonder why Mama never fixed it at home. Why?"

"I've got psoriasis, and eating pork makes it worse. You've got psoriasis now, so don't eat any more bacon. It will make it worse."

"You mean I got this mess from you? Why is it starting now?"

"Yes, it is hereditary. Mine started around my late teens, too. Your grandmother, my mom, had it too. Welcome to the Drennan clan."

"Thanks a lot, Daddy. So, if I just quit eating bacon, it will go away?"

"No, that will help, but you still need to go see a dermatologist to get something to put on it."

The dermatologist peered at my scaly patches, then grabbed his prescription pad. He handed me the prescription for some cream for the spots and some sample tubes.

"Will this make it go away?"

"Yes. But you can't just use this forever. It is a steroid and will make things worse eventually if you use it too long."

"How did I get this, and how can I get rid of it?"

"Psoriasis runs in families. It starts around your age. The problem is the skin. Normally, it takes about a month for cells to move up to the surface. Your skin is doing this in just a few days, making a lot of dead skin cells and scales. It is an inflammatory response. That's essentially all there is to psoriasis. We can take care of the redness and scales, up to a point, but, unfortunately, *there's nothing we can do to cure it.*"

The cream got rid of the scales, but left my skin as white as this paper. Makeup wouldn't cover it. Not much of an improvement, in my opinion. So, I quit using the cream, and the scales came back.

More than 6.4 million Americans suffer from psoriasis, and even millions more around the world have it. It is the second most common skin disease in the United States. It can lead to embarrassment, and this leads to silent suffering in those who have it. Psoriasis is also a leading cause of disability, if you consider that people with psoriasis often become sedentary, due to the lack of energy and associated aches and pains.

Psoriasis is a common skin disease characterized by external local irritations, disorders of the body, and allergies. Psoriatic skin has areas of dry and red scaly spots. The fingernails and toenails have pits. Sometimes the joints hurt, as in arthritis. Many people who have had psoriasis for a while notice a lack of energy.

Inflammation and a thick accumulation of dead skin cells are some of the unsightly, uncomfortable, and even downright painful symptoms that characterize psoriasis. The condition is diagnosed by examining the skin. A tissue sample or blood sample may also be taken and tested to rule out other disorders.

Psoriasis can be aggravated by skin injury; emotional stress; and some forms of infection or irritation, such as cuts, burns, rashes, or insect bites. It can be severe in immunosuppressed people, such as those on chemotherapy treatments for cancer, those with AIDS, or those who have autoimmune disorders, such as rheumatoid arthritis. It is not contagious.

Psoriasis may flare for weeks or months, then subside for a period with no symptoms. But it almost always returns. It sometimes appears on the scalp or the palms of the hands and soles of the feet. Many factors can cause a flare-up of psoriasis, including medications, viral or bacterial infections, obesity, lack of sunlight, sunburn, stress, poor health, cold, and frequent friction. Skin-injury-induced psoriasis is known as the *Koebner phenomenon*.

Psoriasis affects the skin—the soft, smooth, flexible covering of your body. Think of healthy skin as a coat over your bones, muscles, and body organs. This coat has two distinct layers. The epidermis is the outside layer. It is several cell layers thick. Dead cells are constantly being shed from the surface of this layer and are being replaced from below. The dermis is under the epidermis and is made up of a network of collagen and elastic fibers, blood vessels, nerves, fat lobules, and the base of hair follicles and sweat glands.

Psoriasis may cause lesions, patches, or papules (small, solid bumps that do not contain pus) on the surface of your skin. The lesions are usually slightly elevated, can be easily distinguished from normal skin, and are red to reddish-brown in color. The spots are usually covered with small whitish-silver scales that cling to the eruption. If you scrape these scales off, the spot will bleed from tiny points.

You may have a few tiny lesions, or you may have large patches on most of your skin. Usually, your elbows, knees, scalp, and chest are involved. Large areas of the body may be affected in severe cases. The skin over half of the body may crack and bleed. This can be acutely painful, and the body can lose vast quantities of fluid. Secondary infections can set in, and the internal organs can become affected. These infections can progress to cause septic shock and death.

People with psoriasis also have a tendency to get *psoriatic arthritis*. This affects about 10 percent or more of people with psoriasis. This disease leads to pain, swelling, and tenderness of the joints and the tissue around the joints. This type of arthritis is considered to be different from other arthritic diseases.

WHAT CAUSES PSORIASIS?

Psoriasis is a slow and progressive condition that usually first strikes in the teen years, affecting the skin, nails, joints, and one's overall feeling of well-being. It flares up when you become over-stressed, when your skin is injured, or when you develop an allergy. You may notice more scaly spots or that those you have might get worse after you have a systemic infection, like strep throat, or other illness; injure your skin; take a medicine or get vaccinated; deal with a lot of stress; or drink alcohol. Research has shown a link between this condition and the body's ability to properly use fat and create necessary breakdown products. The body needs the breakdown products of fat to lubricate your skin and give you

---

Symptoms of Psoriasis

Psoriasis is a symptom of any of a variety of conditions affecting the body, including allergies, disorders of the immune system, and disorders of the liver. In order to identify psoriasis to find the underlying problem, you must know its symptoms. They include:

- Dry and/or red skin, usually covered with scales.
- Bumpy patches of skin with red borders.
- Pustules, cracked skin, itchy skin, small scaly dots on the skin.
- Aching joints.
- Pitted fingernails and toenails.
- Burning and itching eyes.
- Tiredness and listlessness.

energy. Your body also needs to make the right amount of the right type of hormones to keep inflammation down and your immune system running properly. When your body doesn't produce enough of the proper hormones, your skin suffers. We will discuss this in more detail in Chapter 2.

Heredity also appears to play a role in the development of psoriasis. Millions of psoriasis sufferers can thank defects in genes handed down from their parents for their pain and suffering.

WHO IS AFFECTED BY PSORIASIS?

As mentioned earlier, psoriasis is the second most common skin disorder in the world. It afflicts millions of people worldwide, including more than 6 million Americans. It first strikes most people between the ages of 15 and 35, and 150,000 new cases are diagnosed each year. Sometimes even young children are affected shortly after birth. As mentioned before, there is a very high tendency for it to be shared among blood relatives. Psoriasis can strike anyone, yet it is most frequently found in Caucasians. Men and women are equally likely to be affected.

WHAT ARE THE DIFFERENT TYPES OF PSORIASIS?

The main forms of psoriasis include plaque, guttate, pustular, inverse, and erythrodermic psoriasis.

Plaque Psoriasis

Plaque psoriasis is the most common type of psoriasis. Your skin will have raised, inflamed (red) lesions. These lesions will be covered with silvery white scales made up of dead skin cells. Doctors call this condition psoriasis vulgaris (vulgaris means common). Your knees, elbows, scalp, and trunk are the places to look for this.

At first, the plaque psoriasis lesions look like red dot-like spots and may be very small. These dots slowly grow bigger and become scaly. Scales will come off easily and fall off constantly. If you remove the scales, you will see tiny bleeding points below. This is known as the *Auspitz sign.*

You may have plaques that cover large areas of skin and merge into each other. You also may have lesions in the same place on the right and left sides of your body. You may have psoriasis anywhere on your body, but plaque lesions appear most often on the scalp, knees, and elbows.

These lesions are different in everyone. If you have had psoriasis for a long time, your fingernails and toenails will be affected. The nails will be pitted, scaly, ridged, and/or furrowed. You may become upset, depressed, and embarrassed by the effects of psoriasis on your appearance.

Guttate Psoriasis

When you have guttate psoriasis, you will have small red dots (or drops) on your trunk, arms, and legs. You may have some scales on these lesions. This form can flare suddenly following a streptococcal infection or viral upper respiratory infection. Other events can also lead to an attack of guttate psoriasis, including illness, particularly tonsillitis, a cold, or chickenpox; immunizations; physical trauma; psychological stress; and the administration of antimalarial drugs.

Pustular Psoriasis

Pustular psoriasis causes pus-filled blisters to form on your skin. These blisters are called pustules. The pus is filled with white blood cells; however, this condition is not an infection, and it is not contagious. It might just affect your hands and feet, or it can occur all over your body. Pustular psoriasis tends to cause cycles of erythema (reddening of the skin), pustule formation, and scaling of the skin.

Inverse Psoriasis

You will find inverse psoriasis mainly in your armpit, on your groin area, under your breast, and in other skin folds. It will generally appear as smooth inflamed lesions without scaling. It will become easily irritated by rubbing and sweating.

Erythrodermic Psoriasis

Erythrodermic psoriasis is the reddening of the skin all over your body. Fine scales will fall off. You will also itch severely, and the red areas will hurt. These areas may swell. This form of psoriasis disrupts your body's chemistry and causes substantial fluid, protein, and electrolyte loss. This can lead to severe illness. You can develop edema (swelling from fluid retention) and infection. Your body's temperature regulation can be disrupted. This can also cause an irregular heartbeat or heart attack in people with pre-existing cardiovascular problems. Erythrodermic psoriasis can result in infection, pneumonia, congestive heart failure, and death.

HOW IS PSORIASIS COMMONLY TREATED?

Your doctor will treat psoriasis by trying to clear the lesions from your skin. The treatment prescribed for you will depend upon your type of psoriasis, where it occurs on your body, how severe it is, your age, and your medical history.

Your doctor will usually give topical medications for mild to moderate psoriasis. These medications include:

- Emollients (moisturizers) and lubricants.

- Steroidal creams (cortisone).

- The antipsoriatic drug anthralin.

- Antifungal medications.

- Antibiotics.

- Phenol (a caustic compound generally used as an antiseptic).

- Sodium chloride.

- Various coal tar preparations.

- Vitamin D_3.

You might be told to use these treatments alone, in combination, or with ultraviolet light (UVB). Exposure to sunlight helps clear psoriasis for some people. If you have moderate to severe psoriasis, your doctor will usually prescribe one or more of the following:

• Topical medications listed above for areas of mild to moderate psoriasis focused on control of the symptoms and prevention of secondary infections.

• Ultraviolet B light (UVB).

• PUVA therapy (a combination of psoralen—a chemical that makes the skin sensitive to light—and ultraviolet A light).

• An oral or injected immunosuppressive or anti-inflammatory medication, such as methotrexate (MTX), corticosteroids, or cyclosporine.

• Oral vitamin-A-derived antipsoriatic medications (Tegison and Accutane).

If you have severe psoriasis, you will be given more toxic treatments, such as the systemic drugs hydroxyurea or 6-thioguanine (see Chapter 3 for more information about these treatments). Traditional treatments can stop working for you in the middle of therapy, and you might have to change to another treatment. Many of the topical, oral, and injected treatments given today for psoriasis can cause big problems for you. They can make your skin age rapidly. They can cause skin cancer. You may also have to deal with cataracts, complications secondary to treatments, and secondary skin infections that spread to your internal organs. See Chapter 3 for more about problems caused by conventional treatments for psoriasis.

WHAT IS THE DIFFERENCE BETWEEN PSORIASIS AND OTHER SKIN PROBLEMS?

There are other skin disorders, such as eczema, that also cause skin swelling, skin eruptions, pain, tenderness, and redness. The most obvious sign of psoriasis is excessive shedding of skin cells. These skin cells look like silvery scales on top of the red patches on your skin. Take a look at your fingernails and toenails. If you have psoriasis, you will probably find tiny pits on a few of your nails. Other conditions that can affect your skin are listed below so you can compare your unique condition with these symptoms.

Eczema

Eczema is an inflammatory condition of the upper layers of the skin. Some doctors call it atopic dermatitis. The part of your skin affected by eczema will have patches of blisters, redness, scabbing, and scaling and usually itches. More severe lesions will be redder. The blisters may start weeping fluid. The skin will become thicker after you scratch or rub the patches. Your skin in those areas will be dry.

Rosacea

Rosacea is a flushing or subtle redness on the cheeks, nose, chin, or forehead that comes and goes. If it gets worse, bumps and pimples called papules and pustules appear, and small dilated blood vessels may become visible. The nose may become red and swollen from excess tissue.

Seborrheic Dermatitis

When you have this condition, your skin will have greasy or dry white scales, with or without reddened skin. My infant son had a bad case of this when he was just a few weeks old. He had thick, crusty, yellow scales over his scalp. This condition is called cradle cap in newborns. It can involve the skin on your scalp, face, nose, eyebrows, ears, groin area, and trunk, and behind your ears.

Skin Cancer

Skin cancer causes a change in your skin, such as a growth or a sore that won't heal, or a small lump. Skin cancer growths can vary in appearance. They can appear as shiny, raised growths, or they can be flat. They can begin as a red, crusted, scaly area that doesn't heal, and develop into a wartlike growth. They can begin as small pigmented areas that enlarge over time. They can cause changes in existing warts or moles and the surrounding skin. Never try to rule

out skin cancer on your own. If you suspect skin cancer, see a doctor immediately.

Psoriasis can lead to low self-confidence and self-esteem. It can
cause feelings of embarrassment, anger, depression, and guilt.
Psoriasis is a very common skin condition that most doctors in the
United States and abroad think is incurable. Fortunately, they are
wrong! The Psoriasis Cure has helped to relieve symptoms of psoriasis for many people, allowing them to enjoy normal skin and
active lives once again.

What Causes Psoriasis?

There are standard scientific theories about what causes psoriasis, and there are my findings, found during my research as a biochemist and former psoriasis sufferer, about the causes of psoriasis. This book combines both the beliefs of medicine about what causes psoriasis and my own findings. You are a unique individual, different from everyone else. Your body chemistry is different, the way you live your life is different, and your genetic makeup is different. You will get a better idea of how to control your psoriasis by looking at the principal underlying causes, but your underlying causes may be different from the causes of psoriasis in others you know. Heredity also plays a role in the development of psoriasis—you can thank defects in genes handed down from your mom and dad for your pain and suffering.

This chapter will tell you about the factors that can cause your psoriasis to break out or get worse. These can include stress; an imbalance in your hormones; allergic reactions; toxic substances; the food you eat; and vitamin, mineral, and nutrient deficiencies. This looks like a rather formidable list of factors, doesn't it? Don't let it scare you into giving up on getting rid of your psoriasis. It is easier than you think to get these problems under control. I've already done all the work for you. I've done the research and shown you what's wrong, what's happening in your body, what you need to do, and why this works. Now, all you have to do is take action. When you get rid of the things that are troubling your body, help restore the proper functioning of your glands and liver, and help build up your immune system, you will see dramatic improvement, and perhaps you will even eliminate your symptoms.

STRESS

Stress makes your psoriasis worse by depleting vitamins and minerals that are essential to your health. (See Vitamin and Mineral Deficiencies on page 22.) It weakens your digestive system by reducing the amount of digestive enzymes you make. This makes it harder for your stomach and intestines to properly digest the food you eat. Stress also weakens your adrenal glands, which, among other duties, control inflammation. Long-term stress can overwork your adrenal glands so that they just shut down from exhaustion. If the stress is chronic and severe, your immune system will also suffer.

Your body responds to a complex and tense situation by pouring hormones into your bloodstream. Your pulse quickens, you breathe faster, your blood sugar increases, your digestion slows, and you perspire. Life events have a strong effect on your stress level. If you have experienced stressful life events, you may have noticed a change in your psoriasis symptoms.

Your physical symptoms may begin or become worse as result of your body's reaction to things that mentally or emotionally disturb you. Stress, when properly managed, can work for you as a source of energy. Chapter 8 will suggest ways to help you manage your stress to minimize its impact on your body and, therefore, minimize its contribution to your psoriasis.

HORMONES

Your body relies on chemical messengers called hormones to relay information. These chemicals are made in your endocrine glands. They pour into your blood, then float to specific organs and turn biochemical reactions on or off. Your endocrine glands include the pituitary, the thyroid, the pancreas, and the adrenal glands. (There are others, but for the purposes of this topic, we only need to discuss these.) Read on to find out how too much stress can lead to low adrenal function and chronic fatigue, a shrunken thymus gland and weak immune system, and low blood sugar (hypoglycemia)—all of which are causative factors in psoriasis.

Hormones Secreted by the Adrenal Glands

Your adrenal glands make hormones when you are stressed. There are two adrenal glands in the body—one near the top of each kidney. The inner part of the adrenal gland, the medulla, makes epinephrine (adrenaline) and norepinephrine (noradrenaline). When you are stressed or experience fear, shock, cold, or fatigue, your adrenal glands dump adrenaline and noradrenaline into your bloodstream. These hormones raise your blood pressure and your heartbeat and tell your body to turn glycogen into glucose. They may also negatively affect your psoriasis.

The outer part of the adrenal gland, the cortex, makes steroid hormones, a natural version of the same thing your doctor may have prescribed to stop the inflammation of your psoriasis. So, if your body can make its own cortisone, why would you need to spend your hard-earned money buying more? Prolonged stress makes your adrenal glands work overtime. This will cause your adrenal glands to become exhausted and cease producing cortisone. (Extreme losses of potassium can also cause a depletion of cortisone.) This lack of cortisone contributes to the onset of psoriasis. You will become hypoglycemic (having low blood sugar) when your adrenals get depleted of steroid hormones. Low adrenal function will also cause chronic fatigue. Fatigue, hypoglycemia, and inadequate steroid hormones are common in people with psoriasis.

Hormones Secreted by the Pancreas

The pancreas is a vital part of both the digestive system and the endocrine system. The endocrine portion produces insulin and glucagon. Insulin helps your body use carbohydrates, fats, and proteins and lowers blood-sugar levels. Glucagon has the opposite effect—it raises your blood-sugar levels. Insulin and glucagon work together to help keep your blood sugar steady. If your pancreas isn't working correctly, you can have too little sugar in your blood (hypoglycemia) or too much sugar in your blood (hyper-glycemia, or diabetes). Hypoglycemia is a common problem of people with psoriasis.

When your body is fighting to stabilize blood-sugar levels, it can't focus on proper digestion. Digestion is vital to proper elimination of toxins. If toxins are allowed to build up in the body, they can cause such problems as inflammation and uncontrolled cell division, which, of course, leads to the problems of psoriasis.

You can easily recognize symptoms of hypoglycemia. Are you agitated or irritable when you wake up in the morning or before meals, and then feel much better after eating? Yes? Congratulations! You have just discovered one of the underlying causes of your psoriasis. Now, let's learn more.

Your brain needs glucose to function. If your brain doesn't get enough glucose, you could lose consciousness or even die. Nature keeps this from happening by releasing a chemical called epinephrine, or adrenaline. This chemical sends more sugar into your bloodstream and raises your level back to normal. However, it also aggravates your psoriasis.

Your body and the chemicals in your body react to how and what you eat. You can have too little sugar in your bloodstream if you don't eat often enough, or if you eat lots of sugar or foods that have a lot of sugar in them. Everything you eat eventually gets broken down into a form of sugar in your body. If you don't eat often enough, you won't have a continuous supply of sugar entering your blood.

Have you ever skipped breakfast? Or perhaps lunch? That will give you low blood sugar and release adrenaline into your body. After that, you aren't much fun to be around. You're irritable, agitated, and downright ornery. I control this problem now by eating some form of protein frequently, but while I was pregnant I had a real problem stabilizing my blood sugar. My husband will readily tell you I became "really scary" when I got hungry. He quickly learned to feed me the moment I mentioned hunger, not for my sake, but for his own self-preservation.

Were you a big baby? If so, you might not be able to process glucose properly, since big babies are often a sign of a glucose-processing problem in the mother.

Hormones Secreted by the Thymus Gland

People with psoriasis have problems with their immune systems. Poor immune function certainly appears to be a causative factor in psoriasis. Your thymus gland determines, to a great extent, the health of your immune system. You know your thymus gland has problems if you get frequent infections or suffer from chronic infections. If you have hay fever, allergies, migraine headaches, or rheumatoid arthritis, you probably have something wrong with your thymus gland.

The thymus gland secretes a hormone called thymosin, which regulates the production and maturation of immune cells called T lymphocytes. These white blood cells give you your cell-mediated immunity. This type of immunity is extremely important to help your body fight yeast infections, parasites, and viruses. If you have a viral or yeast infection, your cell-mediated immunity isn't working right. Your cell-mediated immunity also protects you from cancer, allergies, and autoimmune disorders. Thymic hormone levels are typically very low in people exposed to lots of stress, AIDS patients, the elderly, and people prone to infections.

ALLERGIES

Your immune system is your best defense against infection and is highly complex. How does it defend you? It finds "foreign invaders" and sends your white blood cells after them to fight for you. Sometimes, your immune system may think a harmless substance is one of these foreign invaders. This is what happens in an allergic reaction. This mistaken identification will make your white blood cells overreact, and chemicals called histamines are released to fight the substance, which wind up hurting your body, causing the characteristic swelling and inflammation of an allergic reaction. In some people, it appears that an allergic reaction is the cause of their psoriasis.

What are some clues your body gives you that it is having an allergic reaction? Your nose might get congested, you might cough or wheeze, you may itch, you may get hives or other skin rashes, you may have headaches, and you may become fatigued. These are just some possible allergic reactions.

Substances that cause these allergic reactions are called allergens. Anything can cause an allergic reaction. Some of the most common things are pollen; dust; molds; some metals, such as nickel; some cosmetics; lanolin; animal hair; insect venom; some common drugs, such as penicillin and aspirin; some food additives, such as benzoic acid and sulfur dioxide; and chemicals that are in soap and washing powder. Some people are also allergic to certain foods. Common foods that can affect people include chocolate, dairy products, eggs, shellfish, strawberries, and wheat.

There are two types of food allergies. *Cyclic allergies* develop slowly when one eats the same food many times. If you avoid that food for a while, such as four months, you may be able to eat it again as long as you do not eat it too frequently. *Fixed allergies* occur every time you eat a food, for your entire life, no matter how long you wait before eating it again.

Food allergies and food intolerances are not the same thing. If you can't tolerate a food, you can't digest it correctly due to a lack of a certain enzyme or enzymes. This will produce such symptoms as gastrointestinal distress, gas, nausea, and diarrhea after eating the offending food. If you are allergic to a food, your immune system makes an antibody in response to eating it. This will cause the characteristic symptoms of an allergic reaction, including the development of a rash and itching. Some food allergies cause severe reactions, including closing of the throat, difficulty breathing, and possible shock and death. If you can't tolerate a food, you can become allergic to that food because particles of undigested food can get into your bloodstream and cause the allergic reaction.

This is why you really do need to get your immune system and digestion working better by taking the supplements recommended in Chapter 5. After you make your immune system stronger and healthier, you will have less of a problem with allergies.

You never totally get rid of your allergies—you will just minimize the reaction your body has when you are again exposed to the allergen. If you bombard yourself with the offending allergen, your body will have a definite reaction even if your immune system is doing great. So give your poor old body a break—don't make it have to deal with things that cause an allergic reaction if you can avoid it.

TOXIC SUBSTANCES

If your body becomes overrun by toxic substances, your skin will become inflamed and your skin cells will reproduce too fast, leaving behind the pile of silvery scales characteristic of psoriasis. This can happen when your liver isn't doing its job properly, when you don't digest your food properly, when you get an infection, and when you have a food allergy. Toxic substances in your intestines enter your bloodstream through the intestinal wall. Some substances that can do this and hurt you are *Candida albicans* (a yeast-like fungus), bacterial protein breakdown products, allergic reaction byproducts, and free radicals.

Toxic Substances Produced by Your Liver

Your liver filters and detoxifies your blood; however, it can't do its job if it is overwhelmed by too many toxins in your bowels, or if it is damaged. What happens then? All those toxins stay around in your blood and have a party, doing whatever damage they please. Your immune function will be severely compromised if your liver isn't able to do its job. This can lead to psoriasis. The medical establishment has concluded that psoriasis is an immune-mediated disease, because they can treat it with immune suppressive drugs.

Alcohol consumption will make your psoriasis worse because it will increase the absorption of toxins in your gut and impair your liver function. A deficiency in B vitamins makes it very hard for your liver to do its job.

Toxic Substances Produced by Faulty Digestion

Remember from our discussion about your adrenal glands that they produce hormones that slow your digestion when you are stressed? If your body isn't able to completely digest protein, or if your intestines aren't able to absorb protein breakdown products, too many amino acids and polypeptides may accumulate in your bowels. Bacteria in your bowels turn these into toxic compounds called polyamines. Researchers have found lots of these toxic compounds in people with psoriasis. These polyamines prevent your body from making cyclic AMP, regulators of metabolism in the cells. You need cyclic AMP to keep your cells from going crazy and reproducing too fast. When there is a lack of cyclic AMP, the pile of silvery scales, characteristic of psoriasis, accumulates on your skin. Research has also shown decreased levels of polyamines in people with improved psoriasis.

Antibodies from your immune system will bind to a food your body considers a foreign invader to destroy it. This also produces complexes that alter the function of your cells.

Toxic Substances Produced by Infection

Infection, such as candidiasis, can also lead to psoriasis symptoms. *Candida albicans* (a yeastlike fungus) lives in your intestines and doesn't cause harm there. It is a problem when it spreads to other places. It is normally kept under control by your body, but it goes wild when you take certain medications, such as antibiotics, corticosteroids, oral contraceptives, and antacids; when you don't have enough enzymes in your digestive system; or when you eat the wrong things. The yeast can also get into your bloodstream directly or produce toxins that can be even more damaging in your body. It can also decrease your body's production of cyclic AMP, thereby causing your skin cells to reproduce too quickly.

FREE RADICALS

Free radicals are atoms or groups of atoms with at least one unpaired electron. Electrons are negatively charged particles found in atoms. They are usually found in pairs. When unpaired, they are highly reactive and can be very damaging to your body. Free radicals can be produced by exposure to environmental pollution, tobacco smoke, radiation, cooked fats, and alcohol. Your body also produces free radicals naturally when you use energy.

Free radicals are indirect causes of psoriasis in that they can damage your skin tissue and decrease your body's production of cyclic AMP. They also indirectly cause inflammation.

VITAMIN AND MINERAL DEFICIENCIES

You will have red, dry, inflamed, scaly skin if you are deficient in certain vitamins, minerals, and nutrients. You'll also feel tired and listless all the time because your body won't be able to use fat properly. Your skin is fed by your body. If your body isn't working quite right, the skin won't be fed quite right. It won't get what it needs to do and look its best.

Vitamin and mineral deficiencies may be causative factors in psoriasis. Research has shown that people with psoriasis commonly have decreased levels of vitamin A and zinc. The mineral chromium helps regulate your insulin levels. Vitamin E and the mineral selenium help normalize depressed levels of the antioxidant enzyme glutathione peroxidase. (An antioxidant is a substance that fights free radicals.) So, optimal levels of these and other nutrients are needed in the body to help fight psoriasis. Alcohol consumption, malnutrition, and excessive skin cell loss can then further rob your body of nutrients. This lowers levels of the selenium-containing antioxidant enzyme glutathione peroxidase in your body. Stress uses up B vitamins in your body, which, ironically, help combat the effects of stress on the body, so you need to take in more to compensate.

ESSENTIAL FATTY ACID DEFICIENCIES

Everywhere you look, someone is telling you to cut down on the fat you eat. However, certain types of fat are essential to your health. You need some types of fat to feel good and look good— these are called essential fatty acids (EFAs). An imbalance in essential fatty acids can damage your body. Essential fatty acids nourish your body and are the very foundation of your health at the cellular level. They strengthen your cell membranes, help dissolve body fat, increase your metabolism, and increase your energy production. They also help reduce your risk of heart disease and stroke.

Your body needs essential fatty acids to make a group of hormonelike chemicals called prostaglandins, which regulate your inflammatory and immune reactions. Some doctors believe that there is a link between the body's immune response and psoriasis, since inflammation is a characteristic symptom of psoriasis. Some research has supported this belief.

Your problems start when your body makes too much of one type of prostaglandin. Remember when you were a kid and played on a seesaw? What happened when someone heavier than you sat on the opposite side, or you were much heavier than the other person? It wasn't balanced, so you couldn't play. Your body also needs the right balance of prostaglandins.

Some prostaglandins do things that are "good," and some do things that are "bad." Type 1 prostaglandins promote the breakdown of stored fat and decrease inflammation and swelling. Type 2 prostaglandins have the opposite effects—they are involved in allergies and autoimmune reactions and promote inflammation, such as that which produces your red psoriasis lesions. What happens, do you think, when your body makes too much of the Type 2 prostaglandins? You get more inflammation and swelling; more storage of fat; stickier platelets, which lead to heart attacks and strokes; and constricted blood vessels, leading to high blood pressure and kidney disease.

You must obtain essential fatty acids through diet—your body can't make them. A person with psoriasis has a problem getting enough essential fatty acids and making the right type of prostaglandin. So, you need to take essential-fatty-acid supplements to give your body the essential fatty acids you need to form Type 1 prostaglandins.

The Importance of Linoleic Acid

Linoleic acid is the most important essential fatty acid. It is used in your body to make other essential fatty acids, such as gamma-linolenic acid. You can get it by eating seeds, oils, vegetables, and grains. You can seriously reduce your body's ability to properly use linoleic acid by eating the wrong foods and by leading an unhealthy lifestyle—drinking excessively, smoking, etc. What happens if you don't have enough linoleic acid? You will get the red, dry, scaly skin characteristic of psoriasis. This will start first on your face around oily areas and in the folds around your nose, lips, forehead, eyes, and cheeks. You will also notice dry, rough areas appear on your forearms, thighs, and buttocks.

The Importance of Gamma-Linolenic Acid

Gamma-linolenic acid (GLA) is also an essential fatty acid. It helps fight high blood pressure and has important anti-inflammatory properties. Your body needs GLA to make a hormonelike compound called prostaglandin E1 (PGE1), which also has anti-inflammatory properties. Healthy people can make GLA in their bodies by eating foods with linoleic acid, but there are factors that may block the synthesis of GLA in the body. Your body will have trouble making GLA out of linoleic acid if you don't have enough zinc, magnesium, and vitamins C, B_6, B_3, and A in your body. You will also have a problem if you eat too much fat, hydrogenated vegetable oil, and margarine. People with eczema, diabetes mellitus, arteriosclerosis, and psoriasis frequently don't have enough GLA.

If you are deficient in certain nutrients, you have to either eat something that contains GLA, or take it as a supplement because your body will not be able to make it. Do you think the foods you eat right now have enough GLA to support your body's needs? If you've got psoriasis scales on your skin, you don't. Most of the food you eat has been processed by modern methods. These methods take out many of the oils that are essential to your good health. A 1979 study of thirty-eight individuals who took GLA over a period of eight weeks showed the fat-fighting benefits of the oil.

You will find out exactly which supplements you need and what they will do for you in Chapter 5. However, you also need to regulate your diet because prostaglandin production is partially under the control of the hormones insulin and glucagon, and everything you eat affects insulin production in your body. That is why in Chapter 4, you will learn how to change your diet and your life. When your body does not have enough essential fatty acids, you will change sugar to fat much faster than is normal. This will cause your blood-sugar levels to fall quickly, and you will feel hungry all the time.

You now know that stress influences your entire body and can directly and indirectly lead to the inflammation and scales of your psoriasis. Hormones also lead to your skin problems because of their effects on your immune system, digestion, and blood-sugar levels. You also saw how allergies can leave their mark on your skin. Toxic substances can overload your liver, depress your immune function, and lead to skin inflammation and those characteristic skin scales. Vitamin, mineral, and nutrient deficiencies will lead to red, dry, scaly skin and a marked lack of energy. Now that you know what leads to your psoriasis, keep reading to find out how to overcome these problems.

3

The Problems
With Conventional
Medical Treatments

S tandard Western medical treatments for psoriasis can cause a great deal of harm to your body, such as skin irritation, liver damage, and skin cancer. Many are dangerous for women of childbearing age due to their possibilities of producing birth defects. Vital information about the medicines you use and take, such as possible side effects, is often not provided by your doctor or pharmacist. The label on the product often lists only general safety information and doesn't provide detailed information about side effects that can be expected when using the product. Sometimes this information is provided but isn't read by the consumer. Be an informed consumer. Find out everything you can about the products you use and the medications you take.

People infected with HIV often get psoriasis. Unfortunately for them, most of the common treatments for psoriasis, such as corticosteroids, methotrexate, and cyclosporine, will suppress their immune systems. The Psoriasis Cure, shown in Chapter 4, will not suppress your immune system, yet will reduce or eliminate the redness, scales, and other problems you have with psoriasis.

Your medical doctor will treat your psoriasis using either topical treatments—medicines applied to the skin—phototherapy—treatments using light—and/or systemic treatments—medicines taken internally, usually by mouth. These are listed below. The newest method of treating psoriasis is immune therapy. The most popular types of immune therapy are listed with their associated reported side effects at the end of this chapter.

TOPICAL TREATMENTS

Medications put directly on the skin can help clear your psoriasis, but they can also cause a host of other problems in your body. Common treatments and their associated side effects are listed below.

Corticosteroids

Corticosteroids are sometimes prescribed by medical doctors for psoriasis to prevent inflammation. These can cause fluid to build up in your body, bleeding and irritation in your stomach, and confusion. Corticosteroids are usually applied twice each day and are often effective for short-term treatment. If you don't have many psoriasis lesions or spots (less than 10 percent of your body's skin is affected), you might be treated with a high-potency corticosteroid ointment or cream, such as Diprolene (augmented betamethasone dipropionate), Temovate (clobetasol propionate), Ultravate (halobetasol propionate), or Psorcon (diflorasone diacetate). Doctors also use high-potency steroids to treat plaques on the hands or feet. These medications can thin your skin, cause problems inside your body, and make your psoriasis worse. Your skin may atrophy and become discolored. Your adrenal glands can also be suppressed.

Even low doses of corticosteroids can have important long-term effects on your bones. Many patients using topical corticosteroid therapy develop low bone mineral density and eventually osteoporosis (a loss of bone mass resulting from imbalanced bone formation and resorption). Your risk of fracturing a bone is two to five times higher with long-term corticosteroid treatment. Your spine and ribs are affected by corticosteroids more than your neck. This means that if you take corticosteroids over an extended period, you are at greater risk for vertebral fractures. Corticosteroid-induced osteoporosis can occur at any age, even in children. Males and females will lose bone at similar rates during corticosteroid treatment.

You can lose 10 to 20 percent of your bone mass due to corticosteroid treatment. Most bone loss occurs at the beginning of treatment. Your skeleton will be damaged even if you use corticosteroids only infrequently. They damage your bones and interfere with the way in which your body regulates calcium—they decrease your ability to absorb calcium in your intestines, and they increase the amount of calcium that your body excretes in your urine. They directly affect skeletal development by decreasing bone formation and increasing osteoclast-mediated bone resorption. They reduce estrogen in women and testosterone in men, and they inhibit skeletal growth and development in children.

The rate of bone loss is greatest at the beginning of corticosteroid treatment, particularly in high doses. The rate goes down as the dose goes down. Of those taking high doses of corticosteroids, 30 to 50 percent will fracture a bone during therapy. If you take low doses, you will continue to lose bone in your spine at a rate of 2 percent per year.

You can get Cushing's syndrome from long-term use of corticosteroid drugs. Symptoms of Cushing's syndrome are a round red face, obese trunk, humped upper back, and wasted limbs. The skin is thin and bruises easily. The bones become weak and fracture easily. Women become more hairy. Depression, paranoia, and insomnia may become a problem. Approximately one-fifth of people with Cushing's syndrome will develop diabetes mellitus.

The potency of the medication is determined by how much of it enters your tissues and how much it blanches your skin (caused by constriction of the blood vessels). Potencies of common products are listed below. The more potent your medication, the more you are at risk of side effects.

Very-high-potency products include Diprolene AF (augmented betamethasone dipropionate), Temovate (clobetasol propionate), Florone, Maxiflor, and Psorcon (diflorasone diacetate), and Ultravate (halobetasol propionate).

High-potency products include Cyclocort (amcinonide), Diprosone (betamethasone dipropionate), Valisone (betamethasone valerate), Topicort (desoximetasone), Synalar (fluocinolone acetonide), Lidex (fluocinonide), Halog (halcinonide), and Kenalog (triamcinolone acetonide).

Moderate-potency products include Uticort (betamethasone

benzoate), Cloderm (clocortolone pivalate), Cordran (flurandreno-
lide), Cutivate (fluticasone propionate), Westcort (hydrocortisone
valerate), and Elocon (mometasone furoate).

Low-potency products include Aclovate (alclometasone dipropionate), Tridesilon (desonide), Decadron (dexamethasone sodium
phosphate), Cortizone (hydrocortisone), and Cortaid (hydrocortisone acetate).

All of these preparations contain an active ingredient and a solvent. The solvent is a carrier for the corticosteroid, hydrates your
skin, and helps the drug penetrate your skin. Corticosteroid
preparations are available as ointments, creams, gels, aerosols, and
lotions. Ointments get more of the corticosteroid into your
skin. They generally are made with petrolatum, waxes, paraffin,
propylene glycol, or mineral oil. They act as a barrier to prevent
evaporation.

The type of dressing you use to cover the treated area will affect drug penetration. A waterproof dressing will cause your skin
to absorb more medicine. You might also have a reaction to the solvent, in addition to reactions caused by the corticosteroid itself.
Sudden discontinuation of these types of medications can result in
a flare-up of psoriasis.

Some corticosteroid preparations contain antibiotics and anti-
fungals. Neomycin sulfate is the most common antibiotic in these
products. It is available in combinations with several corticosteroids, such as hydrocortisone (Cortisporin), fluocinolone (Neo-
Synalar), and dexamethasone (Neodecadron). Some antifungal
combination products include betamethasone and clotrimazole
(Lotrisone), and triamcinolone and nystatin (Mycolog-II). Greer's
Goo is a mixture of hydrocortisone, nystatin, and zinc oxide generally used for diaper rash, although it is sometimes used in the
treatment of psoriasis.

Calcipotriene

Calcipotriene is a synthetic form of vitamin D_3. It is not the same as
vitamin D supplements. A medical doctor will tell you to rub calcipotriene ointment, such as Dovonex, on your skin twice a day to
control excessive production of skin cells. It can irritate the skin.
You can't use it on your face or genitals. If you use it on large areas

of your skin, you may raise the amount of calcium in your body to unhealthy levels. It is available only by doctor's prescription. Other side effects it may cause are facial irritation, body fold irritation, and worsening of your psoriasis. When you use calcipotriene in combination with UVB phototherapy, your skin is more likely to burn than when UVB therapy is used alone.[1] Other common side effects include itching, burning, dryness, irritation, peeling, redness, and swelling of skin.

Rare side effects of calcipotriene use include abdominal pain; constipation; depression; loss of appetite; weight loss; muscle weakness; nausea; thirst; tiring easily; vomiting; itching, pain, and pus in the hair follicles; and thinning, weakness, or wasting away of skin.

Calcipotriene may increase the chance of kidney stone formation. Another vitamin D derivative, tacalcitol, is currently being evaluated for use as a treatment for psoriasis.

Coal Tar

Coal tar kills skin cells. Manufacturers suggest putting the product directly on your skin. You may have used coal tar bath solutions or shampoo in different concentrations. High concentration products, such as Neutrogena T/Gel, may be irritating to your skin. Coal tar makes your skin more sensitive to ultraviolet (UV) light. It is messy. It does not provide long-term help for most people, it smells strong, and it can stain skin and clothing.

Coal tar contains over 400 compounds, including high concentrations of highly carcinogenic[2] polycyclic aromatic hydrocarbons (PAH). PAHs are absorbed through your skin.[3] Exposure to coal tar may lead to an increased risk of lung, scrotum, and skin cancer.

Anthralin

Anthralin is used to reduce the severity of psoriasis lesions, although it cannot be used on actively inflamed eruptions. In the United States, you can get anthralin only with a doctor's prescription. Your doctor may have given you anthralin ointment, cream, or paste to treat your psoriasis lesions. Anthralin treatment does not usually adequately clear psoriasis lesions. It will irritate your the skin and stain your skin and clothing brown or purple. The stain may last for weeks. Anthralin can cause cancerous tumors. More common side effects are redness or other skin irritation. Some commonly used brand names in the United States are Anthra-Derm, Anthra-Tex, Drithocreme, Dritho-Scalp, and Lasan.

Salicylic Acid

Salicylic acid is used to remove scales. It works better when you use it with topical steroids, anthralin, or coal tar. It causes moderate to severe skin irritation and stinging. Salicylic acid poisoning due to overuse leads to confusion, dizziness, severe or continuing headaches, rapid breathing, and continuous ringing or buzzing in the ears. Studies in animals have shown that salicylic acid causes birth defects when given orally in doses about six times the highest dose recommended for topical use in humans The topical solution is flammable. Breathing the vapors can be harmful to you.

PHOTOTHERAPY

Your doctor may also prescribe ultraviolet light therapy to help reduce the symptoms of your psoriasis. Ultraviolet light (UV) is a form of radiation your eyes can't see. Sunlight is composed of ultraviolet A (UVA) and ultraviolet B (UVB) radiation. Sunlight, UVB, and PUVA (psoralen and UVA) therapies can help clear your psoriasis, but they also can cause a host of other problems in your body. Over your lifetime, ultraviolet rays can cause problems for you, such as cataracts and cancer. Ultraviolet light can damage your eyes by burning your corneas (photokeratitis). Common phototherapy treatments and their associated side effects are listed below.

Sunlight Therapy

Ultraviolet light from the sun can cause injury to your skin. These rays can also cause eye problems. You can't see ultraviolet rays, so you can't tell where they are and how much there is. A lifetime of exposure to sunlight can cause conjunctival, corneal, lens, and retinal damage. Infants and young children have more translucent corneas and lenses, so they are even more susceptible to damage. Sunlight therapy can cause sunburns and can lead to skin cancer. People who are using medication that makes them more sensitive to light, such as psoralen or coal tar, are even more sensitive and at risk of sunburn.

Ultraviolet A (UVA) is the main type of ultraviolet light that reaches the earth's surface through the ozone layer. This is what causes you to tan and burn and produce vitamin D in your skin. Ultraviolet B (UVB) can cause cataracts and skin cancer. Direct sunlight is strongest between 10 A.M. and 3 P.M. UV rays are a greater risk at high altitudes and close to the equator. Snow, sand, glass, concrete, and open water all reflect UV light. You can get increased exposure on your eyes and face from reflection. Artificial sources of UV light, such as welding arcs and sunlamps, can also cause damage to your eyes and skin.

Ultraviolet B Therapy

Ultraviolet B (UVB) rays are short wavelengths of ultraviolet light. UVB rays are used to treat widespread psoriasis and lesions that resist topical treatment. This therapy is administered in a doctor's office with a light panel or light box. You might also be told to use a UVB light box at home. UVB treatment can cause cancer.[4] UVB phototherapy is often combined with other treatments. The Ingram regime consists of a coal tar bath, UVB phototherapy, and application of an anthralin-salicylic acid paste. The Goeckerman treatment consists of the application of coal tar ointment and UVB phototherapy.

PUVA Therapy

UVA rays are long wavelengths of ultraviolet light. PUVA therapy combines UVA light therapy with ingestion of, soaking in, or painting the skin with a medicine called psoralen, which makes your body more sensitive to light. Common psoralen medications include 5-MOP (5-methoxypsoralen), methoxsalen, trioxsalen, and Oxsoralen Ultra (8-methoxypsoralen). Psoralen is taken from certain plants, such as buttercups. These drugs stimulate the production of skin pigment and slow the rate of cell growth.

Side effects of the use of psoralen include nausea, headache, fatigue, redness and blistering of the skin, burning, and itching. It can also cause irregular skin pigmentation if you use it for a long time. It has been found to cause skin cancer when combined with certain medications, such as methotrexate or cyclosporine.

SYSTEMIC TREATMENTS

Doctors will tell you to take a medicine internally if you have a severe form of psoriasis or if more than 10 percent of your body is affected. These can help clear your psoriasis lesions, but they may also have some potentially serious side effects. These medicines and their associated side effects are listed below.

Antibiotics and Antimicrobials

Antibiotics are used to fight streptococcus infection (which can cause psoriasis to break out) and guttate psoriasis. These kill or prevent the growth or reproduction of microorganisms. This means that they not only kill infections that may cause your psoriasis to flare, but they also kill the "good bacteria" in your intestines that help you, and allow the "bad bacteria" to flourish that can hurt you.

This means *Candida* can thrive, and you can get yeast infections after taking antibiotics. Penicillin and ampicillin both have the potential to interfere with the effectiveness of birth control pills. This can lead to unwanted pregnancies. There is an increased possibility of getting physically ill if you drink alcohol and take antibiotics. There is also an increased likelihood of sunburn while taking antibiotics because you become more sensitive to sunlight.

Methotrexate

Methotrexate works by slowing down your cell production and suppressing your immune system. It can cause liver and kidney damage. It can also decrease your body's production of red blood cells (you need plenty of these to carry oxygen in your blood), white blood cells (you need these to fight infection in your body), and platelets (your blood won't clot if you don't have enough in your blood).

Methotrexate works by blocking an enzyme your cells need to live. This causes problems with cell growth. Normal body cells may also be affected by methotrexate. You may experience hair loss. A dose of 4.5 grams has been associated with liver damage, including cirrhosis and fibrosis. Doses of 10 to 25 milligrams per week are often used in the treatment of psoriasis. Methotrexate causes nausea and vomiting in many patients. It may cause birth defects if either the father or mother is taking it at the time of conception or if it is taken during pregnancy. It can also cause harm to or even death of the fetus. It also may sometimes cause temporary sterility.

Some people have developed the Epstein-Barr virus (EBV) during treatment with low doses of methotrexate. In a July 1997 American Medical Association research abstract,[5] it was reported that a patient with psoriasis developed an immune disorder called B-cell lymphoproliferative disorder during long-term treatment with low-dose methotrexate.

Other side effects that may occur with treatment with methotrexate include chills; confusion; dizziness; drowsiness; headache; stomach upset; loss of appetite; difficult and painful urination; dark urine or blood in urine; fever; lower back and side pain; joint pain; swelling of the ankles, feet, or lower legs; unusual bruising or bleeding; cough; hoarseness; blurred vision; sores in the mouth; pinpoint red spots on the skin; red skin; bloody, black stools; bloody vomit; diarrhea; unusual weakness or tiredness; jaundice; and convulsions.

If any of your family members have recently received the oral polio vaccine, you should not stay in the same room very long with them if you take methotrexate. This treatment puts you at high risk of developing polio.

The use of alcohol while taking methotrexate can increase your likelihood of liver damage. Methotrexate will pass into breast milk and enter the bloodstream of a breastfeeding infant. It may impair your ability to drive safely. It may cause photosensitivity—you may sunburn easier and faster.

Hydroxyurea

Hydroxyurea is an antineoplastic agent (a drug used to reduce tumors) that is sometimes used in the treatment of psoriasis symptoms. The exact mechanism by which it is helpful in the treatment of psoriasis symptoms is not known. Hydroxyurea (brand name— Hydrea) might give you anemia and decrease your white blood cells and platelets. No one with any future plans of conceiving or having a child can take it. Hydroxyurea inhibits a cellular enzyme called ribonucleotide reductase, which your body uses to control synthesis of viral DNA. Side effects of its use include neuropathy, nausea, psychiatric disorders, neutropenia (a drop in white blood cells), and nail malformation.

Nonsteroidal Anti-Inflammatory Drugs (NSAIDs)

Nonsteroidal anti-inflammatory drugs (NSAIDs) are used to reduce inflammation. They decrease levels of inflammatory mediators generated at the site of tissue injury by inhibiting the enzyme cyclooxygenase, which catalyzes the conversion of a fatty acid into the inflammatory chemicals prostaglandins and leukotrienes.

NSAIDs bind to plasma proteins, so they can be displaced by or may displace other protein-bound drugs, such as Coumadin (warfarin sodium), methotrexate, digoxin, cyclosporine, oral antidiabetic agents, and sulfa drugs, thus being rendered inactive or rendering these drugs inactive.

Aspirin and ibuprofen can cause stomach upset, bleeding in the stomach, slow blood clotting, and kidney problems. Acetaminophen in high doses can hurt your liver. Aspirin can prolong bleeding time several days after ingestion.

Some of the most common side effects of NSAIDs are constipation, nausea and vomiting, sleepiness, and slowed breathing. Other side effects of NSAIDs may include indigestion, heartburn, loss of appetite, diarrhea, flatulence, bloating, abdominal pain, bleeding, stomach ulcers, kidney failure, and liver dysfunction.

Sulfasalazine

Sulfasalazine (Azulfidine) is often used to treat psoriasis. It suppresses certain inflammatory responses of the immune system. It will suppress your body's production of bone marrow if you use it for a long time.[6]

Cyclosporine

Cyclosporine is used to suppress the immune system. Its side effects include relatively minor symptoms like tremors, headaches, and excessive hair growth, as well as potentially life-threatening conditions, such as high blood pressure, decreased immunity for all kinds of infections, increased cancer risk, and kidney damage.[7] Blood levels of cyclosporine are increased if taken with grapefruit juice.

Patients taking cyclosporine have experienced high blood pressure, kidney damage, seizures, excessive hair growth, excessive gum growth, confusion, coma, and gout. Cyclosporine will cross the placenta to a developing fetus. Pregnant women have reported growth retardation in their fetus, increased rate of miscarriage, and premature delivery.

Though cyclosporine is not currently approved by the Food and Drug Administration (FDA) for the treatment of psoriasis, it is still used to treat it. Other side effects include acne, swelling, fluid in your ankles, cysts on your skin, swelling and fluid in your face, inflammation of your hair follicles, ichthyosis ("fish skin disease"—dry, thick, scaly, dark skin), Kaposi's sarcoma (malignant skin tumors), keratoses (wartlike growths), lymphoma (cancer of lymph nodes and spleen), melanoma (skin cancer), facial papillomas (nonmalignant tumors), purpura (purple or red-brown spots caused by bleeding underneath the skin), vitiligo (loss of pigment in the skin), and flares of dormant lupus erythematosus, herpes simplex, and herpes zoster.

6-Thioguanine

6-thioguanine is an anticancer medication that is sometimes used to suppress symptoms of psoriasis. It can suppress your immune system. It is also toxic to your body.[8] The most common side effect for psoriasis treatment was myelosuppression[9] (when the bone marrow ceases its production of blood cells and platelets).

Retinoids

Retinoids are derivatives of vitamin A. Etretinate is used to treat pustular and erythrodermic psoriasis. Isotretinoin is also used to treat pustular psoriasis. Both can cause birth defects, so women who plan to have children shouldn't take retinoids. Men who plan to father children also shouldn't take retinoids. Etretinate can damage your liver. Tazorac (tazarotene) is a new drug approved by the Food and Drug Administration (FDA) for the treatment of psoriasis. It targets the epidermal cell that produces keratin. Some, however, have reported intense itching and burning on the skin as a result of the use of Tazorac and find that the adverse side effects are just not worth it.

Acitretin

Acitretin is not a retinoid in the true sense of the word, as it is not derived from vitamin A, but it is very similar to vitamin A in its properties. It changes the cells in your skin. Acitretin can cause skin peeling and scaling, hair loss, itching, dry skin, dry mouth, headache, tiredness, impotency, and bleeding gums. Sunlight can increase the severity of the skin side effects. Acitretin can also cause severe birth defects, and there is even some proof that the effect may extend to men who father children. The FDA recommends that women who want to have a child stop taking Acitretin and then wait three years before conceiving.

Acitretin can make the side effects of other drugs worse. These may involve the skin, such as itching around the anus and genitals or even a worsening of psoriasis; headaches; dry mouth; and tiredness. Mild adverse effects involving the hair and mucous membranes have also been reported by patients. It will also cause your lips to become inflamed, cracked, and dry; cause excessive sweating of your palms, soles, and armpits; and make your skin sticky.

Acitretin is used for the treatment of erythrodermic and pustular psoriasis and psoriasis affecting the hands and feet. Acitretin stays in the bloodstream for three to four weeks.[10] Alcohol in your body converts acitretin to etretinate.

Etretinate

Etretinate (brand name—Tegison) can cause dry, peeling skin and lips. It causes birth defects if taken during pregnancy. It is not known how long pregnancy should be avoided after treatment stops to prevent birth defects, but researchers recommend that you never have children if you are treated with etretinate. Patients who receive long-term therapy with etretinate will develop osteoporosis.[11] Etretinate can stay in your blood as long as two years or more after you discontinue treatment. You must never donate blood to a blood bank if you are being treated with etretinate or if you have ever been treated with etretinate.

Vitamin A or any supplements containing vitamin A increase the chance of side effects when taking etretinate. Drinking a lot of alcohol while you are taking this medicine can lead to high triglyceride (a fatty-acid compound) levels in your blood. These can increase your chance of heart and blood vessel disease. Etretinate may also affect blood-sugar levels.

Etretinate may cause dryness of the eyes or excessive tearing in the eyes. If you wear contact lenses, your eyes may be more sensitive while you are taking etretinate and for quite a while after you stop taking it. It can also cause such vision problems as a decrease in night vision, blurred vision, or double vision. This can occur suddenly. Some people who take this medicine may become more sensitive to sunlight than they are normally. It may also cause dryness of the mouth and nose. If this continues, you can get dental disease, including tooth decay, gum disease, and fungus infections. Your psoriasis may get worse with initial treatments.

Other possible side effects may include bone or joint pain or stiffness; dry, burning, itching, red skin; muscle cramps; abdominal pain; unusual bruising; changes in appetite; unusual thirst; extreme fatigue; dark-colored urine; flulike symptoms; jaundice; changes in hearing; earache or drainage of fluid from ear; dizziness; fever; nausea; redness or soreness around and loosening of fingernails; soreness of the tongue; cracking, swelling, or unusual redness of lips; headache; confusion; mental depression; and mood or mental changes.

Isotretinoin

Isotretinoin (brand name—Accutane) has been associated with a 25- to 30-percent increase in birth defects. Defects include malformation of the skull, face, heart, and central nervous system. Side effects include dryness, rashes, and aggravation of psoriasis. If you use isotretinoin with tetracyclines, you may experience swelling of the brain. Any vitamin A supplementation will increase the chance of side effects. Alcohol may cause high triglyceride levels in your blood and possibly increase your chance of harm to your heart and blood vessels.

Isotretinoin can cause your eyes to become dry. This can be a problem if you wear contact lenses. You also may become more sensitive to sunlight than you are normally. It may cause dryness of the mouth and nose. If this continues, you can get dental disease, including tooth decay, gum disease, and fungus infections.

More common side effects include burning, redness, itching, or other signs of eye inflammation; nosebleeds; scaling, redness, burning, pain, or other sign of inflammation of lips. Less common side effects include mental depression; skin infection; peeling of skin on palms of hands and soles of feet; thinning hair; fatigue; pain, tenderness, or stiffness in the muscles, bones, or joints; or rash. Rare side effects include severe abdominal pain, blurred vision or other changes in vision, severe diarrhea, headache, mood changes, nausea and vomiting, pain or tenderness of eyes, rectal bleeding, and yellow eyes or skin.

The most significant laboratory adverse effect was high triglyceride levels in the blood.[12] Patients also experienced increased bleeding during therapy with isotretinoin. Research with pregnant women showed it will cross the placenta and enter the fetal liver and brain.

IMMUNE THERAPY

According to a March/April 1997 research report, researchers now view psoriasis as an autoimmune disease. After researchers noticed that cyclosporine (an immune suppressant) improved psoriasis, they focused their attention on the immune system. The very newest treatments being developed are targeted at specific components of the immune system. These treatments and their associated side effects are listed below.

IL-2 Fusion Toxin

This therapy involves the use of fragments of diphtheria toxin to selectively destroy certain immune cells (those bearing what are termed high-affinity IL-2 receptors). This immune suppressive therapy is considered to be a potential psoriasis therapy because psoriatic tissue contains these IL-2 receptors. It is currently being used on a trial basis for the treatment of psoriasis. Side effects include fever, nausea, flulike symptoms, and rash.

Tacrolimus

Tacrolimus (brand name—Prograf) is derived from soil fungus. It works like cyclosporine as an immune suppressant but is 10 to 100 times more potent on a per-gram basis. Side effects include kidney damage, seizures, tremors, high blood pressure, diabetes, high blood potassium, headache, insomnia, confusion, seizures, neuropathy, and gout.[13] It is currently used to treat liver transplant patients. Animal experiments have shown it can cause miscarriage. Premature delivery may be more common when pregnant women take this drug. Tacrolimus has been reported to cause kidney damage and high potassium levels in the newborn baby, presumably due to its crossing the placenta.

CD4 Monoclonal Antibodies

Researchers believe that activation of the immune cells called CD4 T cells is a primary event in the start of psoriasis. This theory is being studied using vaccines containing antibodies derived from CD4 T cells (CD4 monoclonal antibodies). Treatment at a dose of 140 milligrams intravenously resulted in rashes. Studies are still underway, so no additional side effects have yet been reported.

Physicians currently believe that these medications will slow the progression of psoriasis or eliminate it entirely. None of these medications truly modify your condition—they only lessen the outward signs. These treatments and medications are often expensive and have serious side effects, such as cancer; tumors; birth defects; miscarriage; kidney, liver, and lung damage; diarrhea; and intestinal ulcers.

Conventional medical treatments don't and can't "cure" psoriasis. Doctors treat the symptoms, not the underlying problems. The following chapters will tell you which nutritional supplements you can take to start the healing process and will show you how you can reduce your risk of cancer; kidney, liver, and lung damage; and the multitude of other side effects discussed in this chapter.

4

The Psoriasis
Cure Program

In Chapter 3, you read about all of the unpleasant, sometimes life-threatening, side effects that can occur as a result of the use of standard Western treatments for psoriasis. You don't have to sacrifice your health to get rid of your psoriasis. There is a safer, more natural treatment. This treatment is based on dealing with the root causes of psoriasis and actually healing your body to get rid of your psoriasis, not just hiding or suppressing your symptoms with drugs. People just like you have enjoyed beautiful, smooth, psoriasis-free skin, vibrant health, and a renewed zest for life after following this program. I had a terrible case of psoriasis before I started this program. Now, I enjoy smooth skin and increased energy levels. You have in your hands a way to enjoy this too.

In college, I learned how the body works in courses like anatomy, physiology, and immunology. I learned from my experience with doctors to consider how the body works, even when drugs may be necessary. I learned through my research that vitamins and minerals are extremely necessary for the body to function as it should. I started a protocol of vitamins, minerals, and other nutrients, and my health started showing signs of improvement. I discovered I had allergies that also caused problems with my psoriasis. It took some detective work to uncover all of the problems in my body associated with psoriasis and treat them. Today, my psoriasis problems are only a bad memory.

There's not one magic bullet that will immediately take care of everything. You have to take a comprehensive approach. There are three main parts to this program. The first part involves identification and then elimination of the underlying causes of your psoriasis. The second step is to set up a supplement program. The third part of the Psoriasis Cure Program involves making changes in your diet, lifestyle, and the way in which you deal with stress in your life. Keep reading to find out exactly how you can start treating and curing your psoriasis.

GUIDELINES FOR FOLLOWING THE PROGRAM

So you have decided you really do want to get rid of your psoriasis. How do you get control of your psoriasis? People who have successfully gotten rid of their psoriasis and kept it away follow these guidelines.

Do This for Yourself

Don't do this to please others. You must want to get rid of your psoriasis, to learn what you have to learn, and to do what you have to do to reduce or get rid of your psoriasis symptoms. Don't do this just because someone else wants you to—do it because *you* want to.

Don't Drink Alcohol

Alcohol is a poison and will make your liver work harder to get it out of your bloodstream. If you've got psoriasis, your liver is already sick, so don't make it worse by drinking alcohol.

Don't Expect Sudden Miracles

It is perfectly normal for this program to take a while to start working in your body. You also may see your psoriasis symptoms fluctuate a bit during the initial weeks, as your body starts to heal. If you look closely at your skin every day or several times a day expecting to see immediate results, you might become upset if you don't see the scales fall away. You might panic if you see a slight worsening in the first few days after you stop your prescribed medication, as will happen, or become overconfident when you do notice a definite improvement.

Be Happy With Your Body and Yourself

Have a positive attitude about yourself and about life. Accept yourself the way you are now while you work to improve a little bit every day. Solomon, the wisest man that ever lived, said in Proverbs 17:22, "A happy heart does good like a medicine but a broken spirit dries the bones." Life is all about choices. Choose to be happy.

Be Organized

As the great British World War II leader Winston Churchill said, "Let your advance worrying become advance thinking and planning." Eat foods that are good for you and for your psoriasis at home, and bring your own food along if you need to go someplace where you can't get anything that won't hurt your condition. Arrange your schedule and your life so you have time to eat right without rushing, to exercise, and to do those things most important to you so you minimize stress in your life. Set and achieve your personal goals. Give direction to your dreams. Plan your life expecting positive things to happen.

THE PROGRAM

You are unique, so the program that works for your body will be unique. Your psoriasis did not develop overnight, so don't expect it to go away overnight. You will notice you have more energy within a month. You will probably start noticing considerable improvement in your skin within three months. Your body has to grow new, psoriasis-free skin, and that process takes time, so be patient. Your reward will be that you will feel better and look better than you have in years. That's not just my observation—that is a direct quote from someone who tried this program and was amazed at the results. By the time a whole year has passed, if you have faithfully followed all the steps of this program, you should be enjoying smooth, soft, psoriasis-free skin.

After you have been on this program for a year, begin the maintenance program. You can reduce the amount of supplements you take until you just keep the psoriasis at bay. Chapter 5 will help you with this. If, after you have gotten rid of your psoriasis, you start introducing new ideas or going back to your old ways, you may see a return of your psoriasis. Everything you do and eat will affect your condition. If something makes it come back, stop it. If it doesn't affect your condition, keep it. The rest of your life is a maintenance period. The vitamins and minerals are a *must*. You won't get better without them. The herbs are optional for those who have minor cases. I had a very bad case of psoriasis, so I used the herbs to get better quicker. You can never stop following this program if you want to keep your psoriasis away.

Step 1. Find and Fix Underlying Causes of Psoriasis in Your Body

In the movie *The Wizard of Oz*, Dorothy followed the yellow brick road to find what she was seeking. You need to look beyond your obvious symptoms. You need to understand how your body works. Use what you have learned in Chapter 2 to identify and address your unique underlying problems. As you will recall, these may include:

• Stress.

• Improper function of your hormone-producing glands.

• Allergies.

• Toxic substances in your body.

• Nutrient deficiencies.

Make a concentrated effort to discover your allergies and their causes so you can take the appropriate measures to minimize or get rid of them. Keep in mind that you may also be allergic to the products you use on your skin, such as soaps and lotions. I was surprised to discover that the lanolin found in many creams and lotions, which is believed to be wonderful for softening and moisturizing the skin, actually made my skin break out in a bumpy rash. That rash only got worse when I used expensive lanolin-based creams. I also discovered that vitamin E oil applied externally can cause my sensitive skin to have a bad rash-type reaction. You can get rid of things that may be bothering your skin with the following measures:

- Stop using all the lotions and creams you have been using if they contain lanolin, lanolin alcohol, vitamin E, alpha-hydroxy acids, or aloe vera.

- Use pure olive oil or petroleum jelly to moisturize your skin instead. If your skin is really dry, try wetting your skin with warm water before applying the oil or petroleum jelly.

- After a week or so, when your skin has had time to get over the insult of the offending allergens, try your favorite lotion or cream in a small spot, such as on the top of your hand. Watch for a reaction. It may take a few hours. If your skin hasn't turned red, dry, bumpy, or otherwise reacted to the lotion, it is probably safe to use again.

What can you do to help get rid of your allergies besides boost your immune system? Find the sources of stress in your life and get rid of them. Chapter 8 will help you learn how to deal with the stress you can't get rid of. Chapter 5 tells you which supplements you can take to help your body handle stress, such as vitamin B complex, vitamin B_5, calcium, and magnesium.

You should also rotate the foods in your diet. This means that you should eat different foods at every meal every day for four days, and then repeat the cycle. Never eat the same food more often than once every four days. This will help prevent your body from developing allergies. The Food Allergy Checklist on page 48 will help you figure out which foods cause an allergic reaction in your body. Once you determine the offending foods, eliminate them from your diet. Some primary causes of food allergies are excessive regular consumption of a limited number of foods and

Food Allergy Checklist

Use this checklist to develop a list of suspect foods to help you discover hidden food allergies. Write down how often you eat each of the foods listed below each week. Add up your total for the week. Keep tracking your foods for four weeks. At the end of the period, compile a list of all of the foods eaten four times a week or more. This is your list of suspect foods. Omit them from your diet for one month. Then, reintroduce into your diet one suspect food a day, and note your reactions, if any. In this way, you can determine those foods to which you are allergic.

Food Type	Week 1	Week 2	Week 3	Week 4
Legumes				
Kidney beans				
Lentils				
Lima beans				
Mung beans				
Pinto beans				
Soybeans				
Soymilk				
Tofu products				
White beans				
Condiments				
Catsup				
Gravy				
Jam or Jelly				
Mustard				
Pepper				
Pickles				
Salsa				
Salt				
Soy sauce				

Food Type	Week 1	Week 2	Week 3	Week 4
Dairy Products				
Butter				
Buttermilk				
Cheese				
Cottage cheese				
Cow's milk				
Cream cheese				
Eggs				
Goat's milk				
Ice cream				
Margarine				
Milk shake				
Sour cream				
Yogurt				
Fruits and Juices				
Apples				
Apricots				
Bananas				
Blackberries				
Blueberries				
Cherries				
Coconut				
Cranberries				
Dates				
Dried fruits				
Figs				
Grapefruit				
Grapes				
Lemons				
Melons				
Oranges				
Nectarines				
Papayas				
Peaches				

Food Type	Week 1	Week 2	Week 3	Week 4
Pears				
Pineapple				
Plums				
Prunes				
Raisins				
Raspberries				
Strawberries				
Tangerines				
Grains				
Brown rice				
Buckwheat				
Cold cereal				
Cornmeal				
Millet				
Oats				
Pancakes				
Pasta				
Quinoa				
Rye				
Spelt				
Tapioca				
White flour products				
White rice				
Wheat and whole wheat products				
Meats, Poultry, Fish				
Bacon				
Beef				
Bologna				
Chicken				
Fish				
Ham				

Food Type	Week 1	Week 2	Week 3	Week 4
Lamb				
Liver				
Luncheon meat				
Pork				
Sausage				
Shellfish				
Turkey				
Veal				
Nuts and Seeds				
Almonds				
Brazil nuts				
Cashews				
Hazelnuts				
Nut butter (not peanut)				
Nut milk				
Peanut butter				
Peanuts				
Pecans				
Pistachios				
Sesame seeds				
Sunflower seeds				
Walnuts				
Oils				
Canola oil				
Corn oil				
Olive oil				
Peanut oil				
Safflower oil				
Sesame oil				
Soy oil				

Food Type	Week 1	Week 2	Week 3	Week 4
Sweeteners				
Aspartame (NutraSweet)				
Brown sugar				
Corn syrup				
Fructose				
Honey				
Maple syrup				
Saccharin				
White sugar				
Vegetables				
Asparagus				
Avocado				
Beets				
Broccoli				
Brussels sprouts				
Cabbage				
Carrots				
Cauliflower				
Celery				
Corn				
Cucumbers				
Eggplant				
Garlic				
Green beans				
Kale				
Lettuce				
Mushrooms				
Okra				
Olives				
Onions				
Parsley				

Food Type	Week 1	Week 2	Week 3	Week 4
Peas				
Peppers				
Potatoes				
Radishes				
Spinach				
Summer squash				
Sweet potatoes				
Swiss chard				
Tomatoes				
Turnips				
Winter squash				
Zucchini				
Miscellaneous				
Alcoholic beverages				
Candy				
Chewing gum				
Chocolate				
Coffee				
Cola				
Corn chips				
Flavored gelatin				
French fries				
Fried foods				
Pastry				
Peppermint				
Pizza				
Popcorn				
Potato chips				
Pudding				
Tea				

eating foods that contain lots of preservatives, stabilizers, and artificial colorings and flavorings.

Don't eat any more of the following foods until you know you are not allergic to them:

- Bananas.
- Beef products.
- Caffeine.
- Chocolate.
- Citrus fruits.
- Corn.
- Dairy products.
- Eggs.
- Oats.

- Oysters.
- Peanuts.
- Pork.
- Processed and refined foods.
- Salmon.
- Strawberries.
- Tomatoes.
- Wheat.
- White rice.

If you would like to determine whether or not you are allergic to a certain food, take notice of how your body feels before a meal. Make sure to eat the suspected food with foods that you know do not bother you. Remember, you must eat some form of protein and carbohydrate with each meal. Record your body's reaction after eating a certain food. You will know something is wrong if after eating you get a rash; feel sick or very warm; or have a headache, a rapid pulse, or heart palpitations. Wait at least four hours before eating anything else, as it may take this long or longer for a reaction to occur. If you experience any of these reactions, don't eat the offending food again for sixty days, then try it again in very small amounts. If you get another reaction, don't eat it again. If you experience such reactions as a rapid pulse, heart palpitations, difficulty breathing, or any other potentially life-threatening responses, *do not eat that food again.*

Don't eat things that have artificial colors, such as FD&C Yellow No. 5 dye. Lots of people are allergic to food colorings. I discovered long ago that I got a rash when I drank red Kool-Aid.

My mom thought I was nuts (she couldn't imagine that anything in Kool-Aid could hurt me), but even when I was a preteen, I recognized that anything that had red dye, such as red Kool-Aid, would make me break out—within just a few minutes.

There are other food preservatives and enhancers that manufacturers love to add to foods that can also cause reactions in your body. These include vanillin, monosodium glutamate, BHT-BHA, benzoates, and annatto. Start reading the labels on everything you buy. Ask your waiter at Chinese restaurants if they put MSG (monosodium glutamate) in their food.

Make sure the supplements you take and the products you use are hypoallergenic. Stay away from dust. Use a dehumidifier in your basement. Use paint that has a mold-prevention additive. Don't smoke, and avoid secondhand smoke. Don't take aspirin until three hours after you have eaten. Aspirin makes it possible for more of an allergy-provoking food to be absorbed in your body. You can also buy an air ionizer to purify the air in your home or workplace if you are allergic to airborne things.

Step 2. Take Nutritional Supplements

Promote your healing process with an individualized nutritional supplementation program. As we have seen in Chapter 2, the lack of certain key nutrients can bring on or worsen symptoms of psoriasis. It is, therefore, important for you to know which vitamins, minerals, herbs, and other supplements you need. The appropriate supplements will help heal your liver; boost your immune system; support your glands; improve your digestion; provide your body with energy; and protect your body against heart disease, cancer, autoimmune diseases, skin diseases, and many other diseases, as well as help reduce inflammation in your skin.

Herbs offer you an opportunity to get well and stay well. They help you economically care for your own problems and prevent disease while drug and health-care costs soar. Herbs are a safer, gentler alternative to side-effect-ridden prescription drugs. Herbs sometimes work when Western medical treatments fail. Chapter 5 tells you which herbal supplements will help heal your body and how they will help.

Step 3. Make Changes in Your Life

A healthy lifestyle will improve the quality and quantity of your life. The keys to a healthy lifestyle are:

- Avoiding toxic substances, such as pesticides and cigarette smoke.

- Exercising regularly.

- Learning to manage stress.

- Practicing good sleep habits.

Avoid Toxic Substances

If you smoke, start a stop-smoking program today. Farmers use pesticides, herbicides, and other synthetic chemicals to kill insects and other organisms. Waxes are applied to many fruits and vegetables to keep them looking fresh, but since these waxes don't wash off, the fungicide or pesticide becomes cemented to the produce you eat. Try to buy organically grown produce—produce grown without synthetic chemicals, pesticides, or fertilizers. If you can't do this, ask your grocery store manager where they buy their produce. Foreign produce is more likely to contain excessive levels of pesticides and pesticides banned in the United States. Buy local produce in season. Soak produce in a mild solution of additive-free soap, such as pure castile soap from the health-food store. You can also spray the produce with a biodegradable cleanser from your health-food store, gently scrub it, then rinse it off. Or you can peel off the skin or remove the outer layer of leaves.

Exercise Regularly

Exercise is absolutely vital to help you get rid of your psoriasis. It helps you deal with stress, makes you stronger, helps your body function more efficiently, and increases your stamina and energy levels. Regular exercise also helps you to get rid of tension, depression, worries, and feelings of inadequacy. It will greatly improve your mood. Find something to do that excites you so you will get motivated. Exercise makes you stronger and gives you more endurance. Your whole body will get more oxygen and more nutrients from your exercise. When you exercise on a regular basis, several times a week, you'll find you have more energy. You will more easily be able to achieve your ideal body weight with regular exercise.

Practice Good Sleep Habits

Sleep is absolutely essential to your body and mind. Sleep deprivation will destroy your ability to think. It is a form of torture in Third-World countries. I discovered how effective sleep deprivation is as torture during the first three months of my son's life. I now greatly value a good night's sleep—you should too. It restores your body and refreshes your mind. Try to establish a routine—wake up around the same time and go to bed around the same time every day. Do the same things before you go to bed. This will help you relax so you can sleep better.

Your mind and body become hurt in many ways if you don't sleep enough or sleep well. Conditions such as depression, chronic fatigue syndrome, and fibromyalgia are related to sleep deprivation or disturbed sleep. When your body is deprived of sleep, it releases certain hormones in an attempt to compensate for this lack of sleep. These hormones may worsen the inflammation of psoriasis.

When you have trouble sleeping, find out and fix what is causing the problem. Don't resort to drugs to combat insomnia. First, find out what is keeping you awake. The problem may be mental, such as depression, anxiety, or tension. If that isn't your problem, your food, drink, or medication may be the problem. Keep a record of how you sleep after eating certain foods. If that yummy pizza is causing you to lose sleep, you would be better off without the pizza.

Learn How to Manage Stress

You need to know how to recognize, evaluate, and control stress in your life to get your psoriasis under control. Your body sends out floods of chemicals in response to stress. These chemicals make your inflammation and scales worse and make you irritable and tired. You can't get rid of all your stress, but you can alter the way in which you respond to stress. The stress doesn't determine your body's response—your reaction to stress determines the response. Many things can cause a stress response in your body—a cold draft, driving in heavy traffic, being late for an important meeting, disease, injury, or joy. Learn how to manage your response to stress.

Learn how to relieve stress by calming your mind and body. Easily and powerfully decrease your stress and increase your energy by breathing with your diaphragm. Look closely at your lifestyle. Are you subjecting yourself unnecessarily to stress?

Exercise in some way every day. Follow a stress-reduction diet, such as restricting caffeine, alcohol, and refined carbohydrates and controlling your food allergies. Take the vitamins, minerals, and herbs recommended in Chapter 5 to help your body deal with stress. Chapter 8 will help you manage your stress so you can minimize its impact on your body and, therefore, minimize its impact on your psoriasis.

Eat a Healthy Diet

Hippocrates, the Father of Medicine, said, "Let your food be your medicine and let your medicine be your food." Your diet has a lot to do with your level of health. Scientists have shown that certain dietary practices can cause or prevent disease. Research has also shown that certain foods will immediately help certain parts of your body. You can attain a higher level of wellness by developing and following your own health-promoting diet.

Learn what foods you should and should not eat. Start making this a part of your life from now on. Think of it when you go to the grocery store. Think of it when you go out to eat. No amount of exercise, sleep, vitamins, minerals, or nutritional supplements will make up for eating the wrong things. All of these steps work together as a whole. Read Chapter 7 to learn more about the foods that you should and should not eat to cure your psoriasis.

THE MEDICAL ATTITUDE TOWARD NATURAL TREATMENTS FOR PSORIASIS

Keep in mind that your physician may not listen to your observations about your own body. I once asked a dermatologist if an allergy to certain foods could be aggravating my psoriasis. He asked me where I got such an absurd notion. I told him about my father's warning that pork would worsen my psoriasis. The doctor's reply was, "Is your dad a dermatologist? No? Then he doesn't know anything!" I left his office confused, because I figured he should know about skin conditions since he had gone to medical school and was a dermatologist, but I also knew my dad wouldn't lie to me and had been dealing with psoriasis for longer than that doctor had been alive.

I also knew from my observations of my own psoriasis that when I ate pork products, my psoriasis got worse. The doctor tried to get me to deny my own experience, my own common sense, in deference to his opinion. Don't let your doctor do this to you. Listen to your own good sense. Don't put your total faith in someone just because they are in a position of authority. It is quite easy, safe, and cost effective to remove foods from your diet that aggravate your psoriasis. It is much easier and more productive to listen to your own good sense.

Doctors are fallible. That point was driven very painfully home to me when doctors misdiagnosed my father as having hepatitis when he actually had prostate cancer. By the time they got their act together and actually figured out the real problem, it was too late. The cancer had spread throughout his body. I was forced, by the incompetence of certain doctors, to watch my beloved father die slowly and painfully.

I know very well how it feels to be belittled and ignored by physicians. Let's work together to find and fix the underlying causes of psoriasis in your body. You know your body better than anyone else does.

I have noticed that many doctors can't handle the idea of a natural remedy for psoriasis. I read about a doctor who instead of embracing a therapeutic herb as a remedy that had been proven effective, said that research needed to be done to find out what chemical in the herb produced the desired result, so a drug could be made out of it. That is ridiculous! Why make something unnatural from something natural that works? Why not just keep on using what works—the natural herb itself? Herbs have built-in checks and balances. When you try to extract one chemical, you ruin that balance and get side effects.

The idea of treating an illness with anything but drugs is poorly received by the medical establishment. Alternative natural treatment is such a drastic change from what medical doctors have learned, and many know nothing about these other ways of treating the human body. Many will feel they have to say these alternative treatments are wrong.

These methods of treating your body are not wrong. They are based on a foundation of physiology, anatomy, biochemistry, and immunology. They are also based on the knowledge that we don't know everything there is to know about medicine. We can only find out more and improve how we do things by keeping an open mind.

Medicine is limited and is not an exact science. Not all doctors practice it in a sensible or rational manner. The doctors you have seen for help with your psoriasis prior to reading this book have probably prescribed drug after drug without successful side-effect-free results. You want something better that works. You know you deserve that. This approach looks for underlying causes and helps your body heal itself.

Your body lets you know something is wrong with clues—your symptoms. You shouldn't cover these up with drugs. That will keep you from finding out what your body is trying to tell you. I found that people with psoriasis symptoms usually do have underlying health problems that have gone undiagnosed and untreated. This is a common observation even in medical journals. You should expect more from medicine than a quick dismissal of your problem by giving you the current favorite drug without checking out every possibility.

I tackle my health problems by using the Treatment Triangle. See Figure 4.1 on page 61.

Use the treatment triangle to guide you as you look at your symptoms as clues that there is an imbalance in your body or negative influences from outside your body. Use the clues to help you find and treat the underlying problems in your body. You can use this same principle on any problem you have in your body—people in other countries have been doing it for thousands of years.

Scientific medical research is biased toward drugs. The stan-

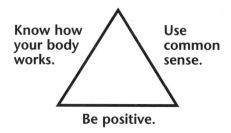

Figure 4.1. The Treatment Triangle.

dard scientific method of proving something works as a treatment is to do a double-blind study. In a double-blind study, a group of people is given a certain treatment and a control group is given a placebo. The placebo is something that is not expected to have any effect, such as a sugar pill. The two groups of people are not told which treatment they are given—the actual therapy being tested or the placebo. Many of the drugs currently used for treatment of certain symptoms have not gone through double-blind studies to prove their effectiveness, yet they continue to be used.

Scientists have been led to believe that this is the only way to prove anything is really useful in medicine. This limits treatments to those that can fit into the double-blind study model, such as drugs. A non-drug-treatment method can help a patient get well and feel better, but if it hasn't been through a double-blind study, it isn't generally accepted in Western medicine. This tunnel vision even extends to treatments that have been used successfully for centuries in other countries, such as herbs, homeopathy, and acupuncture.

Some parts of the psoriasis prevention and cure program, such as taking certain vitamin, mineral, and herb supplements, have been proven effective through double-blind studies. Other parts of the program can't be put into a double-blind format. The change in diet is one of those. It would be impossible to eat certain foods and avoid others without knowing you are doing it. Therefore, the change in diet would not fall into acceptance as a traditional and acceptable form of Western medicine, even if it did great things for your condition. You are living proof that what you eat does affect you, and a change in diet will help your psoriasis. You might be tempted to discount something that could be an effective treatment for your condition if you heard someone from the medical establishment say, "It hasn't been proven." Keep in mind that you know your body better than anyone else does, and you are the best judge of what works for you. If you follow this program and you feel better, you look better, and your psoriasis lesions go away, obviously it works for you.

You deserve to have complete information so you can make your own choice. I wish I had known about this program when I first got psoriasis. I would have never used dangerous drugs as treatment for my psoriasis. Will it work for you? Try it yourself and see. You have nothing to lose but your psoriasis and everything to gain—healthy skin, healthy body, and loads of energy.

How long will this take? You'll start to feel alive again in about a month. It will take about three months before you really start to notice a real difference in your psoriasis. After about a year, you should be trying to remember what your skin used to look like when you had psoriasis. Don't get discouraged. Your patience will be richly rewarded by smooth, psoriasis-free skin, and more energy than you've had in years. Isn't looking great and feeling great worth waiting for?

5

Nutritional Supplements— New Hope for Beating Psoriasis

"It is better to hunt in fields for health unbought,
Than fee the doctor for a noxious draught."

—*John Dryden*

Mother Nature's remedies, such as the leaves, flowers, bark, berries, and roots of plants, are quickly becoming preferred treatment for millions of Americans. They are natural and safe alternatives to dangerous drugs. Vitamins, minerals, and herbal supplements can treat many conditions that drugs can't help. This chapter shows you how to use the right nutritional supplements to take care of your vitamin, mineral, and nutrient deficiencies.

Nutritional supplements are also cheaper than drugs. Insurance companies are starting to take notice. American Western Life Insurance Company and Blue Cross of Washington and Alaska will cover the cost of herbal medicines recommended by your doctor. Even our federal government is intrigued by the possibilities. The U.S. Department of Agriculture spent your tax money on years of studies on plants that have beneficial effects on the human body. The U.S. Food and Drug Administration even said it would welcome any botanical that could treat a problem for which there are currently no effective drugs.

When you start using nutritional supplements, you'll join a

rather large crowd. The *New England Journal of Medicine* says that one in three Americans routinely uses some form of alternative medicine. There are around 4 billion people—80 percent of the world's population—who use alternative medicine right now for their primary health care.[1]

Your body is a self-healing organism. Give your body the opportunity to heal and repair itself, and you'll be rewarded by good health. You will, at the same time, prevent illness. You have seen this self-healing in action—remember the last time you cut yourself? Your cut healed, didn't it? Your body is balanced and can repair itself when your immune system and other defense mechanisms are working properly. When your self-repair systems get overwhelmed or are deficient in something, they need help. This is when you need to use nutritional supplements.

You can find most nutritional supplements in almost all health-food stores, many drug stores, and large supermarkets. The manufacturer's claims for health benefits are generally based on the supplement's use in traditional healing or modern research. Some manufacturers make false promises, so be an informed consumer. Supplements come in many shapes and forms, including tablets, capsules, powders, liquids, creams, and granules. The potency of these supplements will vary, so be sure to read the label to make sure you are getting what you want.

Your body tissues require certain nutrients to function properly. In an ideal world, you would get everything you need for perfect health from the fresh foods you eat. In the real world, however, this is nearly impossible. Due to such factors in the world as chemical pollution and stress, your body needs more nutrients. There are vitamins, minerals, and enzymes that work as substances called antioxidants, which help protect your body from the formation of free radicals. Free radicals are highly reactive molecules that can cause damage to your cells, impair your immune system, and make you susceptible to infection and cancer. Free radicals are also thought to be the foundation of the aging process.

Free radicals are formed in your body by exposure to radiation (overexposure to sunshine, UVA rays, or UVB rays), toxic chemicals such as cigarette smoke, and the process of breaking down stored fat for use as energy in your body. Some nutrients act as antioxidants—free-radical fighters. These nutrients include vitamins A, C, and E, and the mineral selenium. Melatonin, a hormone, is also a powerful free-radical neutralizer. Some herbs have antioxidant properties, as well. You can get some antioxidants from eating certain foods, but in this polluted world, you can't get enough that way to keep up with all the free radicals being made. You can minimize free-radical damage in your body by taking nutritional supplements high in antioxidants. Antioxidant nutrients are among the many recommended for fighting psoriasis in the Psoriasis Cure Program.

Cooking and processing destroys nutrients in the food you eat. This means it is very hard for you to get enough nutrients just by eating food. You need to take in what your body lacks and needs in supplement form. There is a saying, "An ounce of prevention is worth a pound of cure." When you take nutritional supplements, you are implementing preventative maintenance. It's like taking out a nutritional insurance policy on your body. You'll spend much less on medical bills and feel much better immediately.

The vitamins, minerals, and nutritional supplements that will help you reduce or eliminate your psoriasis symptoms, help heal your liver, and boost your immune system, are discussed in this chapter. You'll find out what to take, when to take it, and how much to take.

ESSENTIAL-FATTY-ACID SUPPLEMENTS

Fatty acids are the basic components of fats. Essential fatty acids (EFAs) are termed essential because the body cannot produce them itself, so they must be obtained through the diet. They work with your body to reduce inflammation. Research has shown that psoriasis starts with inflammatory cells,[2] so EFAs will speed healing of your psoriasis. It is extremely important to supplement your diet with these oils because research has shown that blood serum fatty-acid levels are typically abnormal in psoriasis patients.[3] Several double-blind clinical studies have shown that 10 to 12 grams of fish oils added to the diet will result in significant improvement in psoriasis.[4, 5, 6]

In addition to their effects on psoriasis, essential fatty acids improve the condition of your hair, reduce your blood pressure, help prevent arthritis, lower cholesterol and triglyceride levels, and reduce the risk of blood-clot formation and strokes. They help form nerve and brain tissue and help regulate your cardiovascular, immune, and digestive systems. The right amount of EFAs will give you energy without adding body fat. They will act as a magnet and draw oxygen to your cellular membranes. Every cell in your body needs essential fatty acids. They are essential for your body to rebuild and make new cells properly.

The two most well-known groups of essential fatty acids are the omega-3 and the omega-6 fatty acids. The omega-3s include alpha-linolenic acid, eicosapentaenoic acid (EPA), and docosahexaenoic acid (DHA). They can be found in deepwater fish, such as herring, salmon, cod, tuna, and mackerel, and their oils, and canola and flaxseed oils, among other vegetable oils. EPA and DHA are the most active types of omega-3 fatty acids. Alpha-linoleic acid is often found in plants. It is then converted into the active omega-3 DHA in the body.

The omega-6 fatty acids include linoleic acid, cis-linoleic acid, and gamma-linolenic acid (GLA). They can be found in evening primrose oil, black currant seed oil, and borage oil. Gamma-linolenic acid is the most active type of omega-6 fatty acid. GLA tells fat cells in your body called brown adipose tissue to stimulate your metabolism and burn fat. Brown adipose tissue makes up about 10 percent of your total body fat but can burn 25 percent of the calories you consume. Linoleic acid and cis-linoleic acid are converted into GLA in the body. However, if you are stressed, consume alcohol, smoke, have a disease, or eat poorly, this process can be blocked. If these acids are not converted into GLA, they can actually have inflammatory effects. You may need to try a supplement with higher proportions of GLA.

Essential fatty acid supplements must be taken in pure liquid form. Do not heat them. Heat destroys essential fatty acids and can, in fact, create harmful free radicals. You don't need all of these oils, just be sure your source includes both omega-3 and omega-6 oils.

Be careful. Some manufacturers buy essential-fatty-acid oils that aren't the real thing. They lack either the concern or expertise to test it and verify the authenticity and quality of the oil. Be an informed consumer.

Efamol Research Inc., Scotia Pharmaceuticals (Canada) Ltd.

has conducted research for fifteen years on essential fatty acids in their 60,000-square-foot biomedical research facility established in Kentville, Nova Scotia in 1981. You can get abstracts of these studies from their web page on the Internet, or you can get a copy of the full clinical studies by contacting them at 1-888-EFAMOL-1. There are many essential-fatty-acid supplements available from many different manufacturers; however, I would recommend Efamol's products because I have found them to be effective and of good quality.

Scientists in England have also conducted studies on the benefits of sources of essential fatty acids, such as primrose oil, and have found them to be beneficial for skin conditions such as psoriasis.

Fish Oil

You can get lots of omega-3 EFAs from fish oil. Good sources of fish oil include salmon, mackerel, menhaden, herring, and sardines. These have more fat and provide more omega-3 oils than other fish. You will get 3,600 milligrams of omega-3 fatty acids from just four ounces of salmon. Cod can give you only 300 milligrams. Don't rely on cod liver oil as a source of your essential fatty acids. You will overdose on vitamins A and D if you take enough to supply all the fatty acids your body needs. People with diabetes should not take fish oil supplements, due to their high fat content, but should eat fish to get their EFAs.

Flaxseed Oil

Flaxseed oil is rich in omega-3 EFAs, magnesium, potassium, and fiber. It also has lots of B vitamins, protein, and zinc. Flaxseeds have a pleasant nutty taste and can be added to your salad, soup, cereal, or juice. They help reduce inflammation in your body. These oils don't upset your stomach or intestines like nonsteroidal anti-inflammatory medications, such as aspirin, can. Be sure to get extracted, organic, cold-pressed flaxseed oil.

Evening Primrose Oil

Evening primrose oil has the highest amount of gamma-linolenic acid (GLA) of any food substance. It relieves pain and inflammation and enhances the release of sex hormones, such as estrogen and testosterone. Research has proven that it helps prevent hardening of the arteries, heart disease, premenstrual syndrome, multiple sclerosis, and high blood pressure. A 1987 study in the *British Journal of Dermatology* showed participants experienced significant improvement in dry, flaky skin after treatment with evening primrose oil.

Black Currant Seed Oil

Black currant seed oil is rich in linoleic acid and gamma-linolenic acid. It will help protect your body against the negative effects of type 2 prostaglandins, such as inflammation, high blood pressure, and lowered immune function.

Borage Oil

Borage oil is also an excellent source of gamma-linolenic acid. It contains the minerals and essential fatty acids you need for healthy skin and nails. It helps your adrenal glands.

How Much Do You Need?

These oils are available in capsules. You don't need to take each kind of oil—just pick one. My personal favorite is evening primrose oil. If you choose primrose oil to get your body started on the road to health, swallow two whole capsules with a full glass of liquid three times a day at meals; or follow the directions on the bottle of whichever essential fatty acid oil capsules you choose. Don't chew or crush your capsules, and do not take them while you are pregnant. After a few months, you can cut back to two or four capsules a day.

You are the best judge of how much to take. If you can get rid of the redness and scales with just two a day, great. If you need more, try increasing your dosage by one capsule per meal. If within a few days you still do not notice any difference, increase the dosage by another capsule per meal. The only side effect reported from taking too much of these oils was oily skin. If your skin gets oily, just cut back on the amount; however, if as a consequence, your psoriasis gets really bad, or you are experiencing one or more of the risk factors (stress, sickness, an allergic reaction to something), increase the dosage to two capsules three times a day until you get your body and your life situation under control again.

VITAMINS AND MINERALS

Vitamins and minerals contribute to your good health by regulating your metabolism and helping your body release energy from the food you eat. Your body needs small amounts of vitamins and minerals in comparison with carbohydrates, proteins, fats, and water, but those small amounts go a long way. Vitamins work with the enzymes in your body to help keep everything running properly. They also help your body use the carbohydrates, proteins, and fats you eat. You could not break down and use the food you eat without vitamins. Many minerals also serve as coenzymes in the body and are vital to several reactions that occur in the body. When you have psoriasis, your body is deficient in certain vitamins and minerals. You can't get enough of these from the food you eat to overcome your deficiency, so you need to take supplements. Nutritional supplements often work together in their actions, so be sure to take your supplements together.

When purchasing your supplement, make sure the bottle says "sugar, starch, and preservative free," and that the supplement does not contain yeast, corn, salt, wheat, milk, or artificial colors or flavors. Also, check the expiration date. Do not buy a supplement if there is no expiration date or the expiration date is impending, and do not take a supplement once the expiration date has passed. Nutritional supplements are made up of perishable foods, food derivatives, or food byproducts, so their potency can be affected by how long they sit on the shelf of the store and at your home and the temperature at which they are stored.

If you are pregnant, stick with the vitamins your doctor prescribes until the baby comes. Don't start this program while you are pregnant. I know from personal experience that your body goes through monstrous changes during those nine months. Your hormones run wild. These supplements won't do you a lot of good while all that is going on, so just wait until that bundle of joy comes. Then start the program. You'll need the energy it will give you for those late-night and early-morning feedings.

Take a conventional multivitamin/multimineral tablet every day. Use one that provides you with 100 percent or more of the Daily Values, which includes the vitamins and minerals listed below.

- Vitamin A—5,000 international units.

- Vitamin C—60 milligrams.

- Vitamin D—400 international units.

- Vitamin E—30 international units.

- Vitamin K—25 micrograms.

- Thiamine—1.5 milligrams.

- Riboflavin—1.7 milligrams.

- Niacin—20 milligrams.

- Vitamin B_6—2 milligrams.

- Folate—400 micrograms.

- Vitamin B_{12}—6 micrograms.

- Biotin—30 micrograms.

- Pantothenic acid—10 milligrams.

- Calcium—162 milligrams.

- Iron—18 milligrams.

- Phosphorus—109 milligrams.

- Iodine—150 micrograms.

- Magnesium—100 milligrams.

- Zinc—15 milligrams.

- Selenium—20 milligrams.

- Copper—2 milligrams.

- Manganese—2.5 milligrams.

- Chromium—25 micrograms.

- Molybdenum—25 micrograms.

- Chloride—36 milligrams.

- Potassium—40 milligrams.

This will provide you with a baseline for your nutritional supplements. If you have a problem with iron, take a supplement without iron. This is your starting place. You also need to take the additional supplements listed below to provide you with the nutrients in higher dosages to help you overcome your deficiencies and control your psoriasis.

Vitamin A

Vitamin A is essential for healthy skin and nails. It enhances your immune system and helps protect your body from the effects of pollution. A vitamin-A deficiency is common in psoriasis patients.[7] Your skin needs vitamin A for maintenance and repair. It is necessary for healthy cell growth. Your body can't use protein without this vitamin. It is also essential for eyesight. It combines with a pigment called rhodopsin in your retina to give you night vision.

Recent psoriasis research suggests that your T cells are involved in the development of this disorder,[8] and nutritional research has shown that vitamin-A levels in your body affect the normal development of your T cells. Incomplete protein digestion and bowel toxemia are also cited as causes of psoriasis. Vitamin A inhibits the enzyme that turns protein breakdown products (amino acids) into toxic substances called polyamines in your bowels.[9, 10]

Your body must have vitamin A to make bone, tooth enamel, and soft tissue. It also helps keep your skin soft and smooth. It protects your membranes by acting as a scavenger of free radicals in your cells. Free radicals will stick to the vitamin instead of to your cell membranes. This is how vitamin A helps discourage development of abnormal cells, such as are found in breast, stomach, cervical, and lung cancer.

A sign of vitamin-A deficiency is dry hair or skin; rough, scaly skin; fatigue; insomnia; frequent infections; loss of smell and appetite; and dry eyes. A lack of vitamin A will also give you night blindness. Chronic use of mineral oil can make you deficient in vitamin A.

As part of the Psoriasis Cure program, take 25,000 international units (IU) of vitamin A daily for three months, then reduce the dose to 15,000 IU per day. Do not exceed 10,000 IU per day if you are pregnant. If you are taking a multivitamin/multimineral supplement, which I recommend, be sure to include the amount in your multivitamin/multimineral supplement in your calculation of the total amount you ingest. Your multivitamin/multimineral supplement should provide about 5,000 IU. Purchase your individual vitamin A supplements in liquid-filled capsules with 10,000 IU in each capsule.

If you take in too much vitamin A, you will damage your liver. If you have liver disease, don't take more than 10,000 international units (IU) of vitamin A in any form. Vitamin A is a fat-soluble vitamin, meaning it is stored in your fat cells in your liver, so you can overdose with vitamin A. If you get too much, you can cause damage to your red blood corpuscles and get skin rashes, headaches, nausea, and jaundice.

Be sure to take your vitamin A along with other vitamins and minerals because it needs the presence of other nutrients in order to work. You need to make sure you are getting plenty of vitamin E in your multivitamin/multimineral supplement or as an additional supplement whenever you take your vitamin A. A deficiency in vitamin E will keep you from being able to absorb your vitamin A. A deficiency in zinc can also impair your metabolism of vitamin A, so make sure you take your zinc supplement at the same time also. You need to eat protein every day so your body can use the vitamin A you take.

Vitamin B Complex

Vitamin B complex helps your body handle stress and improves all the functions in your cells. It includes vitamins B_1 (thiamine), B_2 (riboflavin), B_3 (cobalamin), B_5 (pantothenic acid), B_6 (pyridoxine), and B_{12} (cyanocobalamin); folic acid; biotin; choline; inositol; and para-aminobenzoic acid (PABA). These vitamins help maintain the health of your skin, hair, nerves, eyes, mouth, liver, brain, and muscles in the gastrointestinal tract. They are also involved in your body's production of energy. You should always take the B vitamins together, but you can take up to two or three times more of one B vitamin than another one for a particular disorder. The B vitamins are a team.

Take up to one vitamin B-complex tablet three times a day with meals to start, then cut your dosage back to one or two tablets a day. Again, it is up to you to decide how much B complex is right for you. Stress increases your need for B-complex vitamins. It is also one of the risk factors of psoriasis. So, if your life gets stressful, take one B-complex tablet three times a day to help your body handle it.

Potencies of B-complex formulations vary, so choose one that has at least:

- Vitamin B_1 (thiamine)—10 milligrams.

- Vitamin B_2 (riboflavin)—10 milligrams.

- Vitamin B_3 (niacin)—50 milligrams.

- Vitamin B_6 (pyridoxine)—5 milligrams.

- Vitamin B_{12}—37.5 micrograms.

- Biotin—15 micrograms.

- Folic acid (or folate)—200 micrograms.

- Pantothenic acid—25 milligrams.

The following B vitamins are to be taken in addition to the B complex.

Vitamin B_1

Your body needs vitamin B_1 (thiamine) for repair and healing of your skin tissue. Vitamin B_1 gives you energy by helping your body use carbohydrates, protein, and fat. It is very important to your nerve cells. It helps your circulation and assists in blood formation. It also helps your brain work better—you will think better and learn better.

Vitamin B_1 acts as an antioxidant by protecting your body from the effects of aging, alcohol consumption, and smoking. If you eat a lot of carbohydrates, you need more thiamine, as it is needed to burn the carbohydrates. Sugar also depletes your stores of thiamine. Don't eat sushi! Raw fish has an enzyme called thiaminase that destroys thiamine. That enzyme is inactivated by heat, such as cooking or boiling. You also need more B_1 during exercise, pregnancy, lactation, and stressful times. Antibiotics, sulfa drugs, and oral contraceptives can decrease the amount of this vitamin in your body.

If you don't have enough thiamine in your body, your thymus gland and lymph tissue will shrink, and you will have reduced antibody response and decreased white blood cell response. You will find thiamine supplements in dosages ranging from 5 milligrams up to 500 milligrams. Your multivitamin/multimineral supplements with B complex included will have between 1 and 10 milligrams of vitamin B_1. Your B-complex supplement will have higher levels.

Signs of deficiency include fatigue, forgetfulness, nervousness, numbness of the hands and feet, tingling sensations, lack of coordination, mental or emotional depression, weakness, and gastrointestinal disturbances. You need magnesium to convert thiamine into its active form in your body, so take your magnesium supplement at the same time. Take one 50-milligram tablet three times a day until your lesions are gone.

Vitamin B_5

Vitamin B_5 (pantothenic acid) helps your adrenal glands produce the right amounts of hormones and relieves stress on the adrenal glands. It is known as the "anti-stress vitamin." Your need for this vitamin increases dramatically whenever you are physically or emotionally stressed or ill. Vitamin B_5 helps your body use vitamins and convert fats, carbohydrates, and proteins into energy. It also helps your immune system by stimulating antibody production. You must have pantothenic acid in order for your body to synthesize cholesterol and corticosteroids. All cells in your body need it. It is necessary for the proper absorption and use of folic acid in your body. Signs of deficiency include nausea, headache, fatigue, and hand tingling.

Take one 100-milligram tablet of pantothenic acid three times a day until your lesions are gone, then take one 100-milligram tablet once a day.

Vitamin B₆

Vitamin B_6 (pyridoxine) helps your body break down and use protein, fats, and carbohydrates. You need more of it when you eat more protein. It promotes healthy skin. Vitamin B_6 affects your physical and mental health. It is necessary for your absorption of fats and protein. It helps keep your sodium and potassium levels balanced, and promotes the formation of red blood cells. It also keeps down infection in your body and reduces the fluid you may have retained. Your body needs it for the synthesis of the nucleic acids RNA and DNA. These hold the instructions for cell reproduction and normal cellular growth. Vitamin B_6 also helps to treat allergies, arthritis, and asthma.

Too little vitamin B_6 will depress your antibody-related and cell-mediated immune function.[11] You can become deficient by not taking in enough B_6 in your diet, eating lots of protein, eating things containing yellow food dyes (which contain hydralazine), drinking alcohol, smoking, or using oral contraceptives. If you suffer from Parkinson's disease, don't take more vitamin B_6 than the amount in your multivitamin—it will inactivate drugs taken for therapy of that disease.

Signs of deficiency include flaky skin, acne, arthritis, anemia, headaches, nausea, a sore tongue, cracks or sores on the mouth and lips, fatigue, oily facial skin, and vomiting. Carpal tunnel syndrome has been linked to a deficiency of this vitamin. Oral contraceptives can increase your body's need for this vitamin. Cortisone drugs block your ability to absorb this vitamin.

Take one 50-milligram tablet of vitamin B_6 three times a day until your lesions are gone. When your psoriasis is gone, you can stop taking extra B_6. If redness or scales return, start taking the vitamin again. If you experience tingling in your fingers, hands, toes, or feet, go down to one 50-milligram tablet a day.

Vitamin B$_{12}$

Vitamin B$_{12}$ (cyanocobalamin) is necessary for carbohydrate, fat, and protein metabolism in your body. It increases your energy. If you don't have enough in your body, you may feel tired all the time. Your tissues that divide most rapidly (such as your blood cells, immune cells, and skin cells) depend heavily on adequate levels of vitamin B$_{12}$. Your body needs it to make enough white blood cells and cells that are normal. Without it, your white blood cells won't be able to do their job—eat and destroy foreign invaders. If you are deficient in B$_{12}$, your thymus gland and lymph nodes will shrink.[12] Your body needs this vitamin for proper digestion, absorption of foods, synthesis of protein, and metabolism of carbohydrates and fats.

Signs of vitamin-B$_{12}$ deficiency include chronic fatigue, depression, digestive disorders, dizziness, drowsiness, eye disorders, hallucinations, headaches, irritability, labored breathing, memory loss, moodiness, nervousness, ringing in the ears, and spinal-cord degeneration. Potassium supplements, anticoagulant drugs, and antigout medications block the absorption of this vitamin in your digestive tract. Large doses of vitamin C can interfere with your ability to absorb vitamin B$_{12}$ from your food, which may lead to deficiency.

Take two timed-release 1,000-microgram tablets a day until your lesions are gone, then take one tablet at least once a week, and more often if you experience signs of deficiency.

Folic Acid

You need folic acid for energy production and the formation of red blood cells. Folic acid will also strengthen your immunity by helping make white blood cells. It is also important for healthy cell division and replication because it functions as a coenzyme in DNA and RNA synthesis. It helps your body use and break down protein.

Signs of deficiency include a sore, red tongue; apathy; digestive disturbances; fatigue; graying hair; insomnia; and weakness. Oral contraceptives and alcohol consumption increase your need for folic acid. Don't take more folic acid than the amount in your multivitamin supplement for a long period of time if you have a hormone-related cancer or convulsive disorder.

Take 400 micrograms a day until your lesions are gone.

The amount of the other B vitamins—B_2 and B_3, biotin, choline, inositol, and para-aminobenzoic acid—in your B-complex vitamin is sufficient for fighting psoriasis.

Vitamin C

Vitamin C is essential for healthy teeth, gums, and bones. It helps heal wounds, scar tissue, and fractures and builds resistance to infection. Your body needs it to make collagen, the "cement" that holds your tissues together. It is also one of the major antioxidant nutrients. Vitamin C also helps to keep your body from turning nitrates (found in tobacco smoke, smog, bacon, lunchmeats, and some vegetables) into cancer-causing substances. The Nobel-Prize-winning chemist Dr. Linus Pauling said vitamin C will decrease your risk of getting certain cancers by 75 percent.

Vitamin C helps your body form skin tissue and helps boost your immune system. It also aids in antistress-hormone production. It has been shown to have antiviral and antibacterial properties.[13] Signs of deficiency include soft, spongy, bleeding gums; poor wound healing; joint pain; dry skin; lack of energy; a tendency to bruise easily; edema; extreme weakness; and pinpoint hemorrhages under the skin.

Disease, stress, steroids, alcohol, analgesics, antidepressants, anticoagulants, and oral contraceptives reduce vitamin C levels in your body. Smoking seriously depletes your store of this vitamin. High doses of vitamin C can cause false-negative readings in tests for blood in your stool. Don't take any medication that contains aluminum at the same time you take your vitamin C supplement. The vitamin makes your intestines absorb aluminum better.

Purchase a timed-release vitamin C supplement containing 100 milligrams of bioflavonoids for every 500 milligrams of vitamin C, as bioflavonoids increase the absorption of vitamin C. Take 2,000 to 10,000 milligrams a day total in divided doses. If you take more than 3,000 milligrams a day, you will need to take a vitamin B_{12} supplement to prevent B_{12} deficiency. If you start experiencing diarrhea, cut back on the dose. When you are well, you don't need as much as when you are sick. Don't take more than 60 milligrams (the Recommended Dietary Allowance) of vitamin C if you suffer from a lack of the enzyme glucose-6-phosphate dehydrogenase. If you do, it could cause rupture of your red blood cells.

Esterified vitamin C is the most effective form. It is made by combining the vitamin C with a mineral, such as calcium, magnesium, or zinc. This makes a form of vitamin C that is not acid and has vitamin C metabolites just like those produced by your body. It gets into your bloodstream and tissues four times faster than regular vitamin C. It also stays in your body longer.

You can irritate your stomach if you take large doses of vitamin C with aspirin. This can lead to ulcers. Don't take more than 5,000 milligrams of vitamin C a day if you are pregnant. Chewable vitamin C can damage your tooth enamel.

Vitamin D

Your body needs vitamin D to heal your skin. Vitamin D is also very important to the bones because the body cannot absorb and use calcium and phosphorus without it. You can also make vitamin D from sunlight on your skin. When you expose your skin to the ultraviolet rays of the sun, a cholesterol compound in your skin is turned into a precursor of vitamin D. Elderly people may be deficient in vitamin D because they may spend little time outdoors in the sun. People with severe psoriasis have been found to have very low serum levels of active vitamin D. Treatment with oral supplements of vitamin D brought the levels up to normal.[14]

Signs of deficiency of vitamin D include loss of appetite, burning in the mouth and throat, diarrhea, sweating on the scalp, insomnia, visual problems, and weight loss. You can also develop hypercalcemia, or too much calcium in your bloodstream, from taking in too much vitamin D in your diet. The long-term effects of hypercalcemia include deposits of calcium in the kidneys, lungs, or arteries.

Mineral oil, steroid hormones, antacids, and some cholesterol-lowering drugs interfere with vitamin D absorption. Liver and gallbladder malfunctions also interfere with the absorption of vitamin D. Thiazide diuretics, such as chlorothiazide (Diuril) and hydrochlorothiazide (Esidrix, HydroDIURIL, and Oretic, among others) interfere with your body's calcium/vitamin D ratio.

Don't take vitamin D without also taking calcium; however, be sure to take your calcium and iron supplements separately. Vitamin D stimulates your intestine to absorb calcium, and calcium and iron compete with each other in your intestine for absorption. This competition can lead to iron deficiency. A vitamin E deficiency will impair the proper metabolism of vitamin D in your liver, so be sure you are getting vitamin E in your multivitamin/multimineral supplement or as an additional supplement.

Take a calcium supplement with vitamin D included—200 IU of vitamin D per every 600 milligrams of calcium. This will also help you obtain the necessary 800 IU of vitamin D per day.

Calcium

Calcium is a mineral that promotes healthy skin. It helps your bones stay healthy and is the cement that holds your cell membranes together. It also regulates muscle contraction and influences your nervous system. Of the calcium taken in your body, 99 percent is stored in your bone. Your body uses this stored calcium to get more for your blood and tissue when needed. It is also involved in the activation of the enzyme lipase, which breaks down fats for use by your body. Calcium helps keep your skin healthy.

You need vitamin D to adequately absorb calcium from your gastrointestinal tract. Stress and lack of exercise can reduce your calcium absorption also. Heavy exercise will interfere with your calcium absorption, but moderate exercise will promote absorption. Iron and zinc can interfere with calcium absorption. Drinking alcoholic beverages, coffee, and soft drinks and eating junk foods, excess salt, and white flour can also lead to loss of calcium. Soft drinks contain lots of phosphate, which interferes with your calcium absorption.

Don't eat too many foods that contain oxalic acid, including almonds, beet greens, cashews, cocoa, soybeans, and spinach, because too much of this acid can inhibit your absorption of calcium. Antacids such as Tums are not recommended as a source of calcium. They do have calcium, but if you take enough to serve as a source of calcium, they neutralize your stomach so there is not enough acid left to dissolve the calcium so you can absorb it. Aluminum-containing antacids can block your body's ability to absorb phosphorus, leading to a deficiency. You have to have sufficient amounts of gastric acid to be able to absorb some forms of calcium, such as calcium carbonate, so don't take large doses of antacids. Calcium citrate has been found to absorb relatively well in people with decreased stomach acid. Some drugs, including cortisone-type drugs, anticonvulsant medications, and thyroid hormone, decrease your intestinal absorption of calcium, so if you are taking any of these drugs or have taken them recently, you need to take more calcium as a supplement.

Signs of deficiency of calcium include aching joints, agitation, hyperactivity, brittle nails, eczema, muscle cramps, nervousness, irritability, high blood pressure, numbness or tingling in the arms and/or legs, rheumatoid arthritis, tooth decay, and a pasty complexion.

Take 1,000 milligrams of calcium along with 500 milligrams of magnesium and 50 milligrams of zinc three times a day with meals. Make sure you also take 200 international units of vitamin D for every 600 milligrams of calcium.

Calcium supplements are more effective when taken in smaller doses spread throughout the day and before bedtime. Calcium will also help you sleep better. Look at the label on the product you choose—don't use one that contains D1-calcium-phosphate. This form of calcium is insoluble and interferes with the absorption of the nutrients in your multivitamin/multimineral supplement.

Take your calcium supplement with a light meal to enhance calcium absorption, but don't drink coffee or other caffeinated beverages with your meal when you take your supplement—caffeine will increase your loss of calcium through your kidneys. You must also watch your phosphorus intake, as too much phosphorus will inhibit your body's absorption of calcium. Try to keep the ratio of your calcium to phosphorus intake at 1 to 1.

Magnesium

Magnesium helps your body use calcium. It also lowers blood pressure and boosts your thyroid gland. Your body needs this mineral to use glucose and fatty acids and to activate amino acids. Magnesium helps your body build new proteins and form cyclic AMP (a regulator of several metabolic processes in the body). Large amounts of calcium can reduce the absorption of magnesium because they share the way they get moved around in the intestine.

Potassium, caffeine, and alcohol increase loss of magnesium into your urine. Eating lots of sugar and high levels of protein will also increase your body's demand for magnesium. Your body needs magnesium to use B vitamins properly.

Signs of deficiency include anemia (from red-blood-cell rupture), loss of appetite, heart rhythm disturbances, anxiety, confusion, depression, disorientation, hallucinations, hyperactivity, irritability, nervousness, restlessness, jumpiness, vertigo, and cold hands and feet. Avoid magnesium supplements if you have kidney disease—you can develop toxic symptoms from excess magnesium if you can't excrete it properly.

Take one combined calcium, magnesium, and zinc supplement tablet containing 500 milligrams of magnesium three times a day with meals.

Your ratio of calcium to magnesium intake should be 2 to 1. When you eat lots of fats (French fries, fried foods, and butter), your magnesium absorption will be reduced because the fat and magnesium make a soaplike compound your body can't use. Folic acid and iron can also increase your need for additional magnesium. You need to take magnesium with calcium and vitamin D because vitamin D stimulates intestinal absorption of magnesium and calcium, otherwise, you'll become deficient in magnesium.

Zinc

Zinc helps your body heal. It is necessary for the proper growth of your skin, hair, and nails. It regulates the activity of your oil glands. It is the most critical nutrient to the health of your immune system, as it is involved in every aspect of immunity. It also protects your liver from chemical damage and is vital for bone formation. Psoriasis has been associated with zinc deficiency or depletion in research studies.[15–18]

Symptoms of deficiency include acne, spotty hair loss, loss of appetite, loss of taste and smell, brittle nails, white spots on nails, scaly skin rashes, frequent infections, impotence and male infertility, irritability, night blindness, poor wound healing, high cholesterol, and fatigue.

Take one combined supplement containing 1,000 milligrams of calcium, 500 milligrams of magnesium, and 50 milligrams of chelated zinc three times a day with meals. Always take zinc in its chelated form; it can cause you to become deficient in copper in its ionic form.

Selenium

Selenium is a powerful antioxidant. It inhibits the oxidation of fats. It protects your immune system by preventing the formation of free radicals. It helps activate your thyroid hormone.[19] Your body needs selenium to make the natural antioxidant glutathione peroxidase. This antioxidant helps reduce inflammation in your skin. Psoriatic patients have low levels of the selenium-containing antioxidant enzyme glutathione peroxidase. You will increase these levels by taking selenium and vitamin E.[20] Selenium supplements will stimulate your white blood cell and thymus function.[21] Your body will have trouble using selenium if you are deficient in vitamin C.

Signs of deficiency include high cholesterol, frequent infections, sterility in men, stunted growth, and poor liver and pancreas function.

Take 200 micrograms of selenium a day. Try to find amino-acid chelate-selenium supplements, such as L-selenomethionine. This is also called organic selenium. Sodium selenate in the same dose will also work.

Chromium Picolinate

Chromium helps your body use cholesterol, fats, and protein. It stabilizes your blood-sugar levels by helping your body use insulin properly. Research has shown that people with psoriasis have high levels of insulin and glucose in their blood serum.[22] Calcium carbonate can impair your body's ability to absorb chromium and lead to a deficiency. Sugary foods and sugar makes you need more chromium. You will become deficient in chromium if your diet is high in refined white sugar, flour, and junk foods.

Signs of deficiency of chromium include fatigue, anxiety, and glucose intolerance (borderline diabetes). Deficiency can also lead to an increased risk of arteriosclerosis.

Take 400 micrograms of chromium picolinate every day with one of your meals or shortly after a meal. Do not take this if you have diabetes, unless directed to do so by your doctor. Stop taking it if you feel lightheaded or get a rash.

HERBS

Nature's medicine chest has been used to help humankind for centuries. Some remedies recommended in the ancient medical text the Egyptian Papyrus Ebers, such as using aloe vera for cuts and burns and mint for digestion, are still used today. Herbs offer you an opportunity to get well and stay well. They help you care for your own problems and prevent disease economically while drug and health-care costs soar. There are effective herbal therapies for a wide variety of problems, such as bruises, swelling, cuts, colds, fevers, minor burns, rashes, menstrual cramps, and flus and other infectious diseases. Herbs overcome the limitations of antibiotics— herbs can be used to treat bacterial *and* viral infections, whereas antibiotics are useless against viral infections. Herbs are a safer, gentler alternative to side-effect-ridden prescription drugs. Herbs sometimes work when Western medical treatments fail. When your liver is even slightly damaged by a toxic chemical, your immune function plummets. Try the following herbs to help heal your liver, boost your immune system, and heal your skin.

Milk Thistle

Milk thistle extract (also known as silymarin) will get your liver to release more bile. It also helps protect your liver, which will keep your blood clean. It prevents free-radical damage by acting as an antioxidant. It is good for adrenal disorders, a weakened immune system, and all liver disorders. Milk thistle has shown value in the treatment of psoriasis.[23]

Silymarin compounds protect your liver from damage and

help rid it of toxins by preventing the depletion of a substance called glutathione. The amount of glutathione in your liver determines your liver's ability to detoxify your blood. The more glutathione in your liver, the more able the liver is in eliminating toxins. Research in double-blind studies has shown it will produce impressive results in improving liver function and removing toxins.[24, 25] Experimental animal studies and human studies have shown that a damaged liver can severely hinder immune function.[26]

Take 300 milligrams of milk thistle three times a day for three months, then take 70 to 210 milligrams three times a day. You are the judge of how much you should take, based on your diet and lifestyle. (If you have damaged your liver by drinking alcohol, you need to take more.)

Echinacea

Echinacea boosts your immune system. It helps your white blood cells and reduces inflammation in your body. This helps you make more T cells, and activates your macrophages (the cells that devour bacteria and other foreign substances that can hurt you).[27] Echinacea fights viruses and works against bacteria by inhibiting the enzymes the bacteria secrete to break through your skin and mucous membranes. If they can't secrete the enzyme, they can't get in your body the way they are accustomed. If you are allergic to daisies, sunflowers, or any plants in the composite family, do not use echinacea.

Purchase a standardized echinacea formulation with 3.5 percent echinacoside. Follow the dosage directions on the bottle. Do not take echinacea for longer than two weeks at a stretch.

Goldenseal

This herb acts as an antibiotic and cleanses your body. It reduces inflammation and kills bacteria in your body. It contains a compound called berberine. Berberine is a broad-spectrum antibiotic. It works against bacteria, protozoa, and fungi such as *Candida albicans*. It is generally nontoxic at the recommended dosage, but it isn't recommended for use during pregnancy, and high doses can interfere with B-vitamin metabolism. Don't use goldenseal for prolonged periods. Use it only under supervision if you have cardiovascular disease, diabetes, or glaucoma.

Take one tablet or softgel three times a day with a full glass of water at meals when you are at risk of infection. Don't take goldenseal for longer than two weeks at a time.

Bilberry

Bilberry is a strong antioxidant. It supports and strengthens the collagen in your skin, reduces inflammation, inhibits bacteria growth, relieves stress and anxiety, and reverses the effects of aging and carcinogens. It helps to control insulin levels in your body. You should note, however, that bilberry can interfere with iron absorption when taken internally.

Follow the directions on the bottle for how and when to take bilberry. The standard dose is 80 to 160 milligrams three times per day. This dosage is adequate for the treatment of psoriasis.

ADDITIONAL BENEFICIAL SUPPLEMENTS

In addition to vitamin, mineral, and herbal supplements, there are several other types of nutritional supplements that are necessary for the treatment of your psoriasis. Read on to learn more about these.

Enzymes

Enzymes have been called the "sparks of life." They play a vital role in all of the activities going on in your body. You need them to digest your food, stimulate your brain, get energy for your cells, and repair your tissues and cells. You couldn't survive without enzymes.

Without the necessary enzymes, carbohydrates, fats, and proteins cannot be digested properly. When protein is not digested completely, amino acids and polypeptides accumulate in your bowels. This partially digested protein can cross through your intestines into your bloodstream. These large molecules can cause an allergic reaction in your body. Incompletely digested protein can also hurt your immune system. Bacteria that live in your bowels turn these partially digested proteins into toxic compounds called polyamines. People with psoriasis have shown increased levels of these toxins.

OK, so your body makes these things called polyamines. So what? Are they really so bad? Yes, they are. Polyamines prevent your body from making cyclic AMP, a regulator of cellular metabolism, which adds to the problem of psoriasis by helping your cells reproduce and grow too fast. If you have psoriasis, your skin cells reproduce and grow too fast. Quite simply put, they grow too quickly to fall off normally, so they stack up and produce those silvery scales.

Research has shown that you have fewer polyamines in your skin and urine when your psoriasis improves.[28] Scientists have also found that the skin of people with psoriasis has too little cyclic AMP and too much cyclic GMP (a regulator of cellular metabolism that works as an antagonist to cyclic AMP).[29, 30] The result of this is your cells go wild and reproduce too fast.

Enzymes will give your stomach and intestines a helping hand. Use one that includes:

- Something to help your body break down protein, such as pancreatic protease.

- Something to break down fats, such as lipase.

- Something to break down carbohydrates, such as alpha-amylase and amylglucosidase.

- Something to break down fiber, such as cellulase and hemicellulase.

- Something to break down milk sugar, such as lactase.

You can get one capsule that contains all these enzymes. Help your body help itself by taking an enzyme supplement every day. Follow the directions on the bottle for when and how to take your supplement. After you get your psoriasis under control, and there are no more outward signs (no redness, no scales, etc.), you can cut back on your dosage. Now, I just take one after a big meal or once a week.

Enzymes are very sensitive to heat and are destroyed when you cook your food. If you want to get enzymes by eating food, you will have to eat raw fruits and vegetables, including pineapples, avocados, papayas, bananas, and mangos.

Garlic Oil

Garlic detoxifies your body and enhances your immune system. It will lower blood pressure and improve circulation. It lowers blood lipid levels. It is used to treat arthritis, asthma, cancer, colds and flu, heart disorders, liver disease, ulcers, and yeast infections. People with depressed immune function, such as those with psoriasis, frequently get candidiasis. Garlic is very effective in fighting fungal infections, such as those caused by *Candida albicans*.[31] It contains many sulfur compounds that give it the ability to heal. If you want odorless supplements, aged garlic (like Kyolic brand) is the best.

Candida albicans normally lives happily in your digestive tract and doesn't hurt anything there. When you take antibiotics, this yeast will go crazy. Your body can absorb yeast cells, pieces of yeast cells, and toxins from these yeast cells. This will compromise your immune system, weaken your resistance, and make you vulnerable to infection.[32] You can treat the condition with natural anti-candida supplements.

Remember the psoriasis risk factors? Stress and sickness are two of them. When you get sick, your body gets stressed. Garlic oil will help keep you healthy. If it was good enough for the people of biblical times (the Egyptians used it to keep their pyramid-building slaves healthy[33]), it's good enough for me.

Take the equivalent to 1,500 milligrams of fresh garlic bulbs a day with a meal. The label on the bottle should state the amount of fresh garlic to which each capsule is equivalent. After you get your psoriasis under control, you can stop taking the garlic. In the areas of your skin that have psoriasis, your cells have 250 to 810 times more free arachidonic acid and a toxic degradation product of arachidonic acid called 12-HETE, than areas without psoriasis. This is due to an inhibitor in your skin in psoriasis areas of the enzyme that usually gets rid of arachidonic acid (cyclooxygenase). Your psoriasis can be made worse by anything that gets rid of cyclooxygenase, such as aspirin and most other NSAIDs. Lipoxygenase inhibitors improve your psoriasis. Garlic inhibits lipoxygenase.

If you are exposed to someone who is sick, or you feel you are coming down with something, take the above-mentioned dose of garlic with every meal until the risk of sickness is over. If you can't stand the smell of garlic, try the enteric-coated tablet. You will need to take at least 10 milligrams of allicin (the active ingredient in garlic) or what is referred to as a total allicin potential of 4,000 micrograms—the equivalent of one clove or 4 grams of fresh garlic every day.

Coenzyme Q_{10}

Coenzyme Q_{10} is a vitaminlike substance that resembles vitamin E in its antioxidant activities. It is sometimes called ubiquinone. It plays a critical role in the production of energy in every cell in your body. It helps your circulation, stimulates your immune system, gets more oxygen to your tissues, and helps reverse the effects of aging. Research has shown that it has the ability to counteract histamine, so it is useful if you have allergies, asthma, or respiratory disease. Signs of deficiency include periodontal disease, diabetes, and muscular dystrophy.

Take one 30-milligram capsule one to three times a day with a full glass of water after a meal. Coenzyme Q_{10} is oil soluble, so you will best be able to absorb it when you take it with oily or fatty foods. Keep your coenzyme Q_{10} supplement away from heat and light. It is perishable and deteriorates at temperatures above 115°F. Get a capsule in liquid or oil form with a little bit of vitamin E added.

Lecithin

Lecithin is a type of lipid that helps your body break down fat and protects your cells. Every living cell of your body needs lecithin. Your cell membranes are largely composed of lecithin. It contains a lot of the B vitamin choline, along with some linoleic acid and inositol. Your body needs choline for the proper transmission of nerve impulses from your brain through your nervous system, for regulation of your gallbladder, and for your liver to function properly. It is used to produce hormones in your body and gets rid of excess fat in your liver by aiding in fat and cholesterol metabolism. It is partly soluble in water, so it will act as an emulsifying agent. Lecithin also helps to give you energy and helps repair damage to your liver.

If you don't have enough choline in your body, your brain function and memory will be impaired. Your level of carnitine (a chemical critical to your ability to burn fatty acids as fuel to make energy) in your heart, liver and skeletal muscle will decline if you are deficient in choline. The drug methotrexate interferes with your ability to absorb choline. Signs of deficiency include high blood pressure, the inability to digest fats (made evident by diarrhea and bloating after eating fats), hypertension, kidney and liver impairment, gastric ulcers, and heart problems. Lecithin can be made from soybeans or eggs. The egg type may work better for people suffering from AIDS, herpes, chronic fatigue syndrome, and immune disorders.

Take one 1,200-milligram capsule three times a day with meals, or use lecithin granules in a dose of 3 grams per day.

THE MAINTENANCE PROGRAM

After you get your psoriasis under control, you won't need to take so many pills. There is a minimum amount that you will need to take, however, to *keep* your psoriasis away. Taking this maintenance level of supplements is critical. If you stop taking them, your psoriasis will come back! In addition to the following recommended supplements, continue taking your multivitamin and multimineral supplement. You must also continue with the other components of the Psoriasis Cure Program, including avoiding allergens and reducing the number of stressors in your life.

Once your psoriasis goes away, you can reduce your dosage of vitamin A to 8,000 to 10,000 IU per day. Take this dose every day. Adults should not take less than this amount unless instructed to do so by a doctor. Continue taking one 30-milligram capsule of coenzyme Q_{10} per day. Try taking two essential-fatty-acid capsules that contain at least 45 milligrams of GLA each a day. Two primrose oil capsules a day keep my psoriasis at bay. You may need a bit more. If you start to see signs of your psoriasis returning, increase your dosage by taking an additional capsule with each meal. If after several days there is no improvement, increase the dosage by another capsule with each meal. You must also continue taking the same dosage of vitamin B complex, selenium, calcium, vitamin D, magnesium, and zinc. Take the original dosage of lecithin whenever you eat very high-fat foods. You do not need to take this every day.

Nutrients work in cooperation with each other in your body. Some nutrients help your body absorb other nutrients. There is a cooperative action between certain vitamins and minerals. They work as catalysts, promoting proper absorption and use of other vitamins and minerals. If you want to correct a deficiency in one nutrient in your body, you need to know what your body needs to best use it so you can take everything you need, not just replace the one thing in which you are deficient. Taking a single vitamin or mineral can be ineffective and dangerous.

You can find nutritional supplements in any vitamin aisle in your favorite grocery store, drug store, or health-food store.

You now know which vitamin, mineral, herbal, and nutritional supplements you need to start reducing the inflammation on your skin, to help your body better deal with stress, to boost your immune system and help your body resist infection, to protect your liver from chemical damage, to help your body break down fat, and to keep your skin healthy.

Doctors and scientists today believe that psoriasis is an immune system disorder. They want to treat you by suppressing your immune system. Why not support it instead by taking nutritional supplements? You can help your body heal itself with this combination of supplements.

As you can see, I've listed a lot of supplements here. You're going to be taking a lot of tablets, capsules, and softgels. Take a good, hard look at your psoriasis and make a commitment right now to do this. It is important that you take the right type and amounts of supplements. Find a reasonably priced source from which to purchase your supplements—you don't need to pay high prices to get good quality products; however, do not sacrifice quality for thriftiness, either. If you find that the brand you are taking does not work for you, switch to a brand of better quality. If you have an adverse effect from taking a supplement, quit taking it.

The vitamins and minerals are a must. Scientific research has clearly established that those with psoriasis are deficient in these nutrients, so you must take them to help your body get rid of your psoriasis. The herbs are optional for those with a minor case of psoriasis.

6

Healthy Habits Really Count

Y ou want to be happy, healthy, and successful. That takes energy. When was the last time you woke up and jumped out of
bed, excited to be alive and looking forward to the day with
anticipation? It's been a while, hasn't it? The same things that are
causing those scales and redness on your skin also leave you feeling drained and sometimes depressed. You don't operate at your
full potential when you have psoriasis. It's hard to be the best you
can be when you don't feel very good deep down inside. After you
have been following the Psoriasis Cure program for a few months,
you'll feel like a great weight has been lifted from you, like the sun
has come out from behind the clouds. You can then work on estab-
lishing healthy habits so you can keep that psoriasis from coming
back again.

This chapter is devoted to showing you what to do to keep
your psoriasis away and to get what you want out of life. You will
learn the importance of making a health-promoting lifestyle, a pso-
riasis-repelling diet, nutritional supplementation, physical care of
your body, and positive attitude part of your daily habits.

You learned in Chapter 4 that there was no magic bullet to get
rid of your psoriasis. However, there are things you can do to start
reducing the outward signs of psoriasis; to reduce your risks of
problems, such as osteoporosis, as a result of standard Western
medical treatments you have received; and to start eliminating

your underlying causes of psoriasis. When you get rid of the underlying problems in your body causing your psoriasis, you will look and feel healthier and have more energy. Use that energy and good health to enjoy the rest of your life on this earth to the fullest. After you get rid of those scales, don't stop there. There's a lot more to life. Keep those scales off by taking charge of your life.

Every day you make choices. You are responsible for choosing a healthy alternative over a less healthy one. Make healthy choices if you want to be well. Your health practices and lifestyle factors incorporate those you learned from your parents, your own habits, and marketing influences. Television, radio, the Internet, magazines, and newspapers constantly bombard you with advice related to your health, diet, and lifestyle. Some of this is aimed not at improving your health but at improving the wealth of the advertiser. Your first step in taking charge of your life and getting and staying healthy is to take personal responsibility for your health. This includes your physical, mental, emotional, and spiritual health. Decide what results you want to achieve. Next, you have to take action. Successful people have one thing in common—they take action.

HEALTHY HABIT #1—LIVE A HEALTH-PROMOTING LIFESTYLE

You can keep your psoriasis at bay, improve the quality of your life, and extend the time you have on this earth by living a healthy lifestyle. This includes getting regular exercise, maintaining good sleep habits, and not smoking. Life is full of choices—choose to engage in physical activities that you like, choose not to smoke, and choose to make a good night's sleep important in your life.

Exercise

Have you chosen a sedentary activity, such as watching television, over some form of exercise because you felt you didn't have the energy? After you start following the Psoriasis Cure Program, you won't have that excuse anymore. Don't think you have the time? If you have time to watch a movie or read the paper, you have the time to exercise. Are you not motivated? Find something to do that excites you so you will get motivated. Exercise makes you stronger and gives you more endurance. Your whole body will get more oxygen and more nutrients from your exercise. When you exercise on a regular basis several times a week, you'll find you have more energy. Instead of making you more tired, exercise will make you less tired. You'll more easily be able to achieve your ideal body weight with regular exercise.

Do you feel restless, tense, depressed, or run down, or do you have trouble sleeping? Scientific studies have shown that people who get regular exercise feel better about themselves, are happier, and sleep better. Exercise also gets your body to release substances called endorphins. Endorphins greatly improve your mood, in the same way morphine does. So, the next time you are feeling low or stressed, don't wallow in self-pity or take a drug to get a high— exercise, and you'll get a natural high.

Exercise can help you live longer, but if you're not used to exercising, or if you have heart problems, you need to see a physician before you start putting increased demands on your heart.

If you are healthy enough to start exercising now, choose several things to do that you will like. Commit yourself to doing one of those activities every day for at least twenty minutes. An hour is better. This can be anything from bowling, gardening, golfing, Jazzercise, stair climbing, tennis, walking, or anything else you like to do that gets your heart beating faster. You want to get your pulse rate going a bit higher than it is when you are resting. Aerobic exercises, such as brisk walking, jogging, bicycling, cross-country skiing, swimming, dancing, and racquet sports, are the best ones to strengthen your heart. If you don't have comfortable athletic shoes that fit well, get some before you start.

Learn how to check your pulse so you can make sure you are exercising enough to get some benefit, but not so much that you may cause harm. Put your index and middle finger on the side of your neck below your jaw. Feel for your carotid artery and check your pulse. Count your heartbeats—the number of times you feel the pulse—for six seconds, then multiply that number by ten. That's your pulse rate.

OK, now you know how to check your pulse—but what is good, and what is bad? To figure out what your exercising pulse should be, subtract your age from 185. This number is the upper limit of your safe exercising pulse range. Then subtract 20 from your upper-limit figure. This figure is the lower limit of your optimum safe exercising pulse range. Make sure your pulse rate remains within this range when you exercise. Stop and rest if your pulse rate starts to go above it. For example, if you are 40 years old, subtract 40 from 185 (185 − 40 = 145). Then subtract 20 from 145 (145 − 20 = 125). Your pulse rate should remain between 125 and 145 while exercising.

Do something different every day so you don't get bored. If you like being around other people, find a friend or several friends to exercise with you. Start out slowly, such as exercising just ten minutes a day, and work up from there.

Heart Health

It is very important to have your doctor give you a physical evaluation before you undergo an exercise program to ensure that your body is in good health. Many conditions, particularly heart and respiratory disorders, can prevent you from beginning a program of exercise without a doctor's supervision. If you have any of the following symptoms or risk factors, it is possible that you have a heart disorder, and you should first get your doctor's permission before beginning any exercise program. Consult your doctor if you:

- Smoke.
- Have high blood pressure.
- Feel extremely breathless after physical exertion, such as climbing a few stairs.
- Feel pain in your chest, arms, teeth, jaw, or neck during or after exercise.
- Feel dizzy, faint, or lightheaded during or after exercise.
- Feel weak or fatigued during or after exercise.
- Have heart palpitations or an irregular heartbeat.
- Have any known heart conditions.

Sleep

Your mind and body become adversely affected in many ways if you don't sleep enough or sleep well. Conditions such as depression, chronic fatigue syndrome, and fibromyalgia are related to sleep deprivation or disturbed sleep. When you have trouble sleeping, you should find out what is causing the problem, and fix it. Don't resort to drugs to combat insomnia. First, find out what is keeping you awake. The problem may be a mental or emotional one, such as depression, anxiety, or tension. If that isn't your problem, your food, drink, or medication may be the problem. (See the inset "Insomnia" on page 98.)

Sleep is necessary to give the body a rest. During this period, the entire body slows down. This gives the body an opportunity to repair itself and to discard wastes that accumulated faster than the body could dispose of them during the day.

There are five stages of sleep. These stages can be separated into two categories: rapid eye movement (REM) sleep and non-rapid eye movement (non-REM) sleep. Stages 1 through 4 can be categorized as non-REM sleep. Stage 1 is the stage of lightest sleep and stage 4 is the stage of deepest sleep. REM sleep is a lighter stage of sleep than stage 3 or 4. Your brain is most active during your REM sleep stage. You usually go into REM sleep about ninety minutes after you fall asleep. REM sleep is the stage in which dreams occur.

Sleep occurs in cycles, in which the sleeper goes through each stage of sleep, generally in order from stage 1 to stage 4 to REM sleep, although the cycle does not always follow this order. REM sleep is very important for physical and mental health, as one must enter each stage of sleep in cycles for restful sleep. Scientific studies have shown that people deprived of REM sleep demonstrate profound personality changes, such as extreme irritability, depression, and anxiety. These problems disappear when they are allowed to get REM sleep.

I discovered the truth of this personally after having a baby. Because of the demands and needs of my new baby, I didn't get REM sleep for three months. Since it takes about ninety minutes before the brain goes into REM sleep, and the child never gave me more than forty-five minutes at a stretch to rest, I never got a

---

Insomnia

Insomnia is a sleep disorder in which the affected person has difficulty falling asleep or staying asleep through the night. It is actually a symptom of an underlying problem rather than a disease in and of itself. Some common causes of insomnia include depression; anxiety; stress and tension; brain function disorders; physical pain and discomfort; drug abuse and dependence; and certain foods, drinks, and medications.

---

chance to go into REM sleep. I (and everyone around me at that time) can vouch for the accuracy of the description of a person deprived of REM sleep. Don't do that to yourself. You won't feel good, and you won't be able to function very well. Think of a good night's sleep as one of the nutrients critical to your good health.

Don't Smoke

Smoking is the leading cause of death in America because it is the most important risk factor in cancer and heart disease, the two leading causes of death. Smokers get cancer and heart disease three to five times more than nonsmokers do. A smoker will die seven to eight years sooner than a nonsmoker. Cigarette smoke has more than fifty cancer-causing chemicals. If you want to feel good, look good, and be healthy, you must not smoke. Life is all about choices. Choose not to smoke. Are you afraid that you can't do it? Who is in control of your life—you or those little rolls of tobacco?

Want some help? Here are some ways you can stop smoking:

- Get a piece of paper and a pen and write down all the reasons you want to quit. Read these to yourself out loud every morning when you get up and when you go to bed at night.

- Pick a deadline—a day you will never again touch a cigarette. Tell ten of your friends that is the day you will quit.

- Take action! Meet your deadline.

- Get rid of all ashtrays, matches, cigarettes, and butts.

- Find something else to do with your hands and mouth, such as playing with your pencil or chewing gum, fruit, or raw veggies.

- Tackle your problem like you would eat an elephant—one small piece at a time. Focus on getting through today. Don't worry about tomorrow until it is here.

- Join the crowd—40 million other people in America have quit smoking, so you can too.

- Use the power of visualization. It works for businesspeople and professional athletes—it can work for you too. Close your eyes and imagine how you would look with unstained teeth; how you would enjoy the full flavor of great-tasting food; how fresh your breath would smell; how great your clothes, car, and house would smell; how you would spend your extra money; and how great it would feel to be in control of your life.

- Call the American Cancer Society and ask where the nearest support group meets. Join it.

- Feeling stressed? Use relaxation techniques such as deep breathing to relax instead of grabbing a cigarette.

- Don't go places that make you think about smoking.

- Reward yourself for your accomplishments every day, such as by buying yourself something you want with the money you would have spent on cigarettes.

HEALTHY HABIT #2—EAT A PSORIASIS-REPELLING DIET

In Chapter 7, you will learn what you should and should not eat in order to make your psoriasis go away and keep it away. Start making these practices a part of your life from now on. Think of it when you go to the grocery store. Think of it when you go out to eat. It takes about twenty-eight days to make something a habit. Starting today, for the next twenty-eight days, write down what you ate at the end of each day. Was it good for your psoriasis, or bad for you? What should you do differently tomorrow? No amount of exercise, sleep, vitamins, minerals, or nutritional supplements will make up for eating the wrong things. All of these things work together as a whole.

HEALTHY HABIT #3—TAKE SUPPLEMENTS

You learned about the supplements you should take in Chapter 5. These vitamins, minerals, herbs, and nutritional supplements will help to heal and maintain the health of your body naturally. These are nontoxic dietary supplements; they are not drugs. They work over time to nourish your body and replenish what it needs to promote healthy skin. What you do in the next sixty days will set the stage for your personal results.

These supplements are just that—supplements to a healthy diet. You can't make up for unhealthy habits, such as smoking, not exercising, eating unhealthy foods, and having a negative attitude by popping a few pills. You do need to make taking supplements a part of your everyday life because you are deficient in several things, and you need to boost your immune system, but look at your life as a road you are traveling. For the long haul, if you really want good health and a feeling of well-being, you must devote your attention to ongoing development of a positive mental attitude, a healthy diet, and a regular exercise program.

HEALTHY HABIT #4—TAKE GOOD PHYSICAL CARE OF YOUR BODY

You must take good physical care of your body if you want to be healthy. This involves wearing the proper clothes, practicing deep breathing exercises, maintaining good posture, receiving massages, and exercising. Exercise was covered above, so we'll just talk about the others here.

Select natural fibers, such as cotton, linen, silk, and wool, for your clothes. Wear only cotton, linen, or silk materials in the summer. Man-made fibers, such as rayon and polyester, do not allow perspiration to evaporate. If your perspiration stays on your skin, bacteria will grow. Those bacteria can cause a rash on your skin and will make your psoriasis worse.

Learn to breathe deeply, naturally, and easily using your diaphragm. Your body will have more energy and be less stressed when you breathe deeply. Feeling sleepy in the middle of the day? Take a few deep breaths. You'll become more alert immediately. When you breathe this way, you'll also make your spine more erect, push your shoulders back, and pull your head up—this will improve your posture. Make deep breathing one of your daily habits.

Maintaining good posture is extremely important as one of your healthy habits. When you are slouched and slumped, with your head down, you force yourself to breathe shallowly, not from your diaphragm, and you make yourself tired and sore. You can force your vertebrae out of alignment and cause muscle spasms. The next time you feel low, nervous, or scared, let your body tell your mind to perk up by assuming a more energetic posture. It will send a message to your subconscious that you are ready to rock and roll. Make a habit of paying attention to the way you are holding your body and the way you are breathing. The next time you feel really beat, notice the positioning of your head and shoulders and how you are breathing. Give yourself a quick boost by straightening up and breathing deeply. If your muscles feel tight when you straighten up, you may benefit from massage.

There are many massage techniques, ranging from gentle to very vigorous. Massage can help relieve tension in your muscles and help you relax. Find a good therapist to give you a massage when your muscles are very tense. They quality of the massage is related more to the skill of the therapist than to the type of massage.

HEALTHY HABIT #5—DEVELOP A POSITIVE ATTITUDE

The real foundation of great health is a positive mental attitude. Your daily thoughts and your emotions have a great effect on your quality of life and your health. The Bible says in Phillipians 4:8, "Whatsoever things are true, honest, pure, lovely, of good report; if there be any virtue, any praise, think on these things." You may not be able to control some things that happen in your life, but you can control how you respond to life events. Your attitude determines how you will view and respond to your life challenges.

Want to be happier, healthier, and more successful? Adopt a positive mental attitude. It is essential to boost you to be the best you can be.

Your attitude, like your physical body, needs attention to stay fit. You won't become physically fit after just one exercise session—you have to make exercising a habit. You have to make maintaining a positive mental attitude a habit too. Work at being positive and optimistic throughout your life.

Bad things will happen to you, but it isn't those things that happen in your life that determine your direction in life; it's your response to those challenges that will shape the quality of your life. Think about your life so far. Haven't your failures sometimes led to success? Haven't your disappointments, heartbreaks, and hardships led to compassion, joy, and ecstasy? Direct your mind toward positive things, so that you can experience better health and more happiness in your life.

Psychologist Abraham Maslow studied healthy people over a period of more than thirty years. He discovered that healthy people progress up the steps of the pyramid of human needs. You have to meet your needs at the bottom of the pyramid before you can go to the next level. As you meet your needs, you move closer to health and well-being.

Maslow's Hierarchy of Needs is as follows: physiological needs, safety, love, esteem, self-actualization. Your primary needs— hunger, thirst, sexuality, and shelter—must be met before you can go to the next step. These are basic survival, essential biological, or physiological needs. After you get those under control, then you need security, order, and stability in your life. You need to feel safe so you can deal with the world. After you feel safe, you can love and be loved. After love comes self-esteem, including feelings of approval, recognition, and acceptance. The last step, the top of the pyramid, is self-actualization—using your creative potential for self-fulfillment.

Maslow found that self-actualized people had similar characteristics. Look at what he found, and start making these qualities part of your daily life. Self-actualized people:

• Appreciate the basic pleasures of life, such as nature, children, and music, with wonder, pleasure, and awe every day.

- Have a mission in life—a problem outside themselves that requires their creative energies. The mission is unselfish (not just accumulation of wealth) and is ethical and philosophical.

- Find solutions to problems, rather than feeling sorry for themselves.

- Perceive reality more effectively than other people and are more comfortable with it. They are objective about their own limitations, strengths, and possibilities. They use this to clearly define their values, goals, desires, and feelings. Uncertainty doesn't frighten them.

- Accept themselves, others, and nature. They accept their own shortcomings without condemning their faults. They are able to feel guilt, shame, sadness, anxiety, and defensiveness when necessary but don't experience them to unrealistic degrees. They have a sense of right and wrong, and when they feel guilty, they do something about it.

- Are spontaneous in their personal lives, thoughts, and impulses. They are not nonconformists, but they don't let convention keep them from doing something they consider important or basic.

- Need privacy and have a quality of detachment. They are self-governing and enjoy being active, responsible, self-disciplined, and decisive. They hate being helplessly ruled or used by others.

- Have times when their intense emotions transcend themselves. They experience a feeling of unlimited power, a loss of place and time, and great wonder and awe.

- Have deep feelings of sympathy and affection for, and identification with, other people, even when occasionally angry, impatient, or disgusted with those people.

- Have deeper and more profound interpersonal relationships than many other adults, yet not deeper than a child's relationships. They have a small circle of friends and deep ties with just a few individuals. They are kind and patient with just about everybody, but they do tell hypocritical, pretentious, pompous, or self-inflated people what they need to hear.

- Are friendly toward people of all races, colors, classes, political beliefs, and educational levels. They are aware of how little they know related to what they could know and what others know, and that they can learn something from everyone.

- Are very moral and ethical.

- Have a good sense of humor but don't laugh at jokes that hurt others. They like spontaneous thoughtful humor.

- Are very imaginative and creative. They are resourceful when solving problems.

Start on your road to self-actualization by taking charge of your own positive mental state, your life, and your health. You can then direct your own life. Commit yourself to being the best you can be at whatever you do. There is genius, power, and magic in boldness. The seven steps you can follow on your road to self-actualization are discussed below.

Be Optimistic

Optimism is necessary if you want to achieve ideal health. It helps prevent disease and works on healing your body. Pessimism can seriously hurt your health. Optimists are healthier, live longer, and have fewer and less severe diseases. Your level of hope or hopelessness and how much you make permanent and universal explanations for your troubles relates to how much you will suffer from stress, anxiety, and depression. If you don't have much hope, you will tend to collapse when things go wrong. When something bad happens to you, don't blame yourself and lower your self-esteem. This doesn't mean you shouldn't take personal responsibility, it just means you shouldn't beat yourself up every time something goes wrong. If you are a pessimist right now, learn how to be optimistic. Make thinking with a positive attitude a daily habit so you can be healthier and happier and enjoy life at a higher level.

Listen to Your Self-Talk

You constantly talk to yourself in your head. Your subconscious hears and responds to this. What are you saying to yourself right now? Is it positive or negative? Drive out all negative self-talk. Replace it with positive self-talk. You can use questions and affirmations to do this.

Ask Questions of Yourself That Help

Your brain will answer every question you ask. The quality of your life will equal the quality of the questions you make a habit of asking yourself. What questions do you ask yourself when you come upon an obstacle or problem? Do you ask yourself self-esteem crushing questions, such as "Why does this always happen to me?" or "Why am I so stupid?"? Today, start making a habit of asking better questions, such as "What can I do to make this a better situation?" or "What can I learn from this so it won't happen again?"

If you are depressed, you may ask yourself, "Why am I so unhappy?" or "Why does everything go wrong for me?" Replace these questions with "What do I need to do to get more energy and be happier and more energetic?" After you answer that question, ask yourself, "If I were very happy with lots of energy right now, how would I feel?" Questions can be very powerful in your life. These questions will reprogram your subconscious to believe you are very happy. If you have eliminated physical reasons for depression, such as vitamin and mineral deficiencies, your subconscious will start believing you are happy, and your depression will evaporate.

Try making a habit of asking yourself the following questions every day.

- What do I need to do today to reach my goals?

- Who do I love the most? Who loves and cares for me?

- What do I feel strongly enough about in my life to commit myself to? Why do I want to be committed to that?

- What do I enjoy most in my life now?

- What am I grateful for in my life and why?

- What makes me most excited in my life? Why?

- What makes me the most happy when I think of it in my life right now? Why?

Good questions will give you a new and improved attitude. Ask better questions if you want to have a better life.

Use the Power of Positive Affirmations

Your subconscious mind will be influenced by your affirmations— statements declared as facts with some emotional intensity behind them—to create a healthy positive self-image in you. I *will* eat right. I *will* exercise. I *will* get rid of my psoriasis. You can fuel the changes you want in your life with positive affirmations. Create your own affirmations. Phrase your affirmations in the present tense. See it already come true in your mind. Make your affirmations positive. Don't use negative words, such as not or never. Try to feel the positive emotions that your affirmation generates. Keep your affirmations short and simple yet full of feeling. Make your affirmations personal and meaningful. See yourself experiencing what you are affirming. Now, stop for a minute and write down five affirmations. Recite these out loud when you drive, shower, pray, or at other times you are alone.

Create Success by Setting Positive Goals

Positive goals are powerful ways to build self-esteem and build a positive attitude. Your goals have the power to bring maximum happiness and the highest possible success. Goals can create a cycle of success. When you reach the goals you have set, you will feel better about yourself. This good feeling will help you reach your other goals. Always work toward a program of personal goals. Take action—nothing will ever happen without action. Make sure your action is constructive, leading to worthwhile consequences. Become more goal conscious, and make goal-setting a habit. Give direction to your dreams.

Your human nature makes you yearn to achieve, accomplish, and attain. Set goals that light a fire of enthusiasm within you and kindle the flame of your imagination so you can enjoy happiness and deep rewards from your daily life. The following guidelines will help lead you from wish to fulfillment. Keep an open mind and be patient. You are what you are today because of your choices in response to events that have occurred over time. Changes in your habits and attitudes will take time. Goal-setting has always been and always will be the most important ingredient in self-motivation and successful achievement. You not only need to know what to do, but you must also know why you do it because you are a unique individual, and you must be able to make independent decisions.

Get into the "do it now" habit. Make your goals practical and action oriented. Use techniques to stay involved in progressive constructive action. Use as many of your five basic senses (sight, hearing, smell, taste, and touch) as you can when you learn, to help you retain your new knowledge. Hold written text in your hand. Read it out loud. Listen to yourself as you read. You will have more difficulty remembering something you heard than remembering something you read, so be sure to look at the written words. Write down your goals. The act of writing uses your sense of touch. You will get results far more quickly when you use the three basic senses of sight, hearing, and touch than you could achieve using just one of these.

You learn by repetition. Spaced repetition is one of the most effective forms of learning. Go over your goals every day. Invest in yourself and your success. Your goals will help you grow as a person and achieve greater success. You must define your idea of success in meaningful terms if you want to use your unique talents and abilities to conquer your challenges. Develop a plan of action to clarify your priorities and take you systematically toward your goals.

Find a time of day to think about and work on your goals that works best for you. Set a regular schedule for this, some time you can work without interruption. You won't become truly great by accident, nor will you achieve success by a quirk or fate or a stroke of fortune. You must take action. Get a piece of paper and write down five goals you plan to accomplish tomorrow. Do this every day for five days. Every day, record your successes (those goals you accomplished). Ignore the things you didn't get done. You can work on those tomorrow. Build success habits by recognizing the joy of success. See how powerful positive action, as opposed to self-punishment, is toward producing success? You have just taken action toward forming goal-setting habits and attitudes. Turn thoughts into action. Actions lead to habits. Start now to create and follow your plan of action every week.

- List things you want that you can easily achieve. This will give you some little victories and build your confidence in your ability to achieve more difficult objectives.

- Keep working on your list. Make it as long as you like. List all of your wants and wishes. List immediately tangible wants or needs and long-range goals, such as providing for your child's education. Dare to dream. Don't judge yourself by your past experience and your present abilities, but do make your goals attainable and realistic within your physical limitations. You never stop learning, growing, or living. Plan for what you will become. Don't back off from things you want because you feel unworthy.

- Be clear and specific. If you aren't making the kind of progress you want and are capable of making, you need to more clearly define your goals. You must know exactly what you want to achieve.

- Don't use any negative words in your stated goals. State your goals in positive terms.

- Use the present tense, not the future tense, when you state your goals. You must believe you have already reached your goal if you really want to reach it. This will program your mind to achieve the goal. See yourself as you will be when you have achieved the goal, and feel like you will feel when you have achieved the goal.

- Set short-term goals to help you achieve your long-term goals. Ask yourself every day what you need to do that day to achieve your long-term goal.

Remove your mental self-limiting restrictions so you can develop more of your potential. Think of the elephant as an example of the way in which your mind, and sometimes only your mind, can hold you back. A baby elephant is tied to a small post to keep it in one place. It tries and tries to pull free but can't because it isn't strong enough. After a while, it accepts the fact that it can't get free, so it stays in place. A grown elephant is also held in place by a small rope and a small post. It could easily pull up the post from the ground and run away, but it doesn't. Why? It thinks it can't. The elephant's mind is really the only thing holding it to that post. Don't let your mind keep you tied to your limitations. You mold and make your destiny. You have unlimited potential except for the limits you put on it. Ponder on the promise of Matthew 7:7: "Ask and it will be given to you, seek and you shall find, knock and it will be opened to you."

Use the Power of Positive Visualization

You can live your dreams by using the powerful tool of visualization. See your life the way you want it to be in your mind before it happens. Picture yourself in ideal health. Focus your creative powers on your goals. You can move from where you are now to where you want to be by using your mind. Dream of what you want to achieve, then shift to realistic and objective thinking and planning. Use your creative mental power of visualization to turn your plans into reality.

Picture ideas, events, circumstances, and even concrete objects coming to fruition in your mind. You do have the ability to do this, even if you are not used to it. Language is based on visualization. Words represent an object or an action that you see. Some words express complex thoughts. If you can talk and write, you can visualize.

Visualization enhances your ability to achieve. It is much more than idle daydreaming. It consists of clear and distinct pictures of the result that will come from the pursuit of your goals. Use as many of your senses as you can in your mind. See, feel, taste, touch, and smell. See the picture vividly and sharply so you can describe it to others to help them see it as clearly as you do. The picture of yourself in possession of your goals stimulates your desire, puts a fire under your creativity to help you plan action, and motivates you to *take* action. It helps to relieve stress caused by doubt, uncertainty, and fear of the future because you will have already seen the future. Make a plan to use visualization as a tool to reach your goals. This will activate your personal potential for success by linking your creativity and your ability to take logical actions. See the roadblocks you will run into on the way to your goal and see how you find creative solutions to overcome them. Experience the future now through visualization. That will help you to know what to expect and how to make your desired future come true. Make visualization a habit. Develop your ability to visualize through consistent daily practice.

Use the Power of Laughter

Life will be much more enjoyable and fun for you if you laugh often. Laughter enhances your immune system and improves your physiology. It helps your blood flow to your extremities better and improves your cardiovascular function. It helps your body release natural mood-elevating and painkilling chemicals called endorphins. It helps move oxygen and nutrients to your internal organs.

You can have more laughter in your life by learning to laugh at your shortcomings or mistakes, learning how to use humor when it is appropriate, finding a comic strip you like and reading it every week, watching something funny on television, renting a funny video or going to see a funny movie with a friend, learning how to laugh and play from kids, and finding something funny in an uncomfortable situation.

Take care of yourself by making a daily habit for the rest of your life of getting enough exercise, eating the right foods, taking the right supplements, getting enough of the right kind of sleep, and greeting every day with a positive attitude. Take charge of your life. You're worth it, so give yourself the best.

The Anti-Psoriasis Diet

You've probably heard the saying, "You are what you eat." This is true. The food you eat can make you more healthy or less healthy; it can strengthen or weaken you. It can make a disease worse, or it can get rid of symptoms of a disease. In this chapter, you'll learn how to fuel your body's healing process with foods that can lessen your psoriasis symptoms and perhaps even help prevent some of your symptoms. The result will be a decrease in the external signs of psoriasis and an increase in the health of your skin and body systems. This change will be psychologically satisfying as well because you will be able to judge the results by your mirror.

This isn't a stringent diet, based on just a few foods. That type of diet won't work for you long term, because you and I know you won't stick to it indefinitely. You need something that is easy to follow. That's why this program is sensible, flexible, and easy to follow. You'll need to stay away from certain foods, but you can still enjoy a lot of the things you love. You will need to eat foods low in saturated fats, high in essential fatty acids, and high in antioxidant nutrients. Focus on whole, unprocessed plant foods. You can eat vegetables to get fiber.

GUIDELINES FOR FOLLOWING THE ANTI-PSORIASIS DIET

How do you get control of your psoriasis? People who have successfully gotten rid of their psoriasis and kept it away follow these guidelines:

- *Never skip a meal.* If you're a bear when you get hungry, you probably have low blood sugar. When you skip a meal, you are likely to eat too much when you do eat, and you will probably not choose the best foods for your condition. You'll crave fatty, sugary foods. Eat healthy, and eat often.

- *Keep an eye on the types of fat you eat.* Don't eat anything that is fried. Stay away from hydrogenated oils. (Throw out that margarine!) Once your oil is cooked, it is bad news for your psoriasis. Add butter or oil to your food *after* it is cooked. Use just water to cook it. One of the easiest and most effective ways of helping your psoriasis is to limit your intake of saturated fats and hydrogenated oils.

- *Don't "diet."* A strict diet is a burden for you, and you'll quickly drop it for something easier. You'll do much better if you follow a flexible, easy plan that includes healthy foods you enjoy.

- *Be organized.* As mentioned in Chapter 4, eat foods that are good for you and for your psoriasis at home, follow the guidelines for eating out on page 113, and bring your own food along if you need to go someplace where you can't get anything that won't hurt your condition.

EAT TO BEAT PSORIASIS

Eating healthfully is one of the most important things you can do to get healthy and stay healthy. Research has shown that there is a special connection between food and your psoriasis symptoms. Some foods can help reduce the inflammation and scales, while other foods can help prevent the appearance of symptoms.

You now know that the three-step Psoriasis Cure Program includes eating foods that help you get rid of your psoriasis and avoiding certain foods. The powerful anti-psoriasis diet includes foods containing antioxidants, foods with bioflavonoids, foods

Guidelines for Eating Out

The tips in this chapter may be useful when cooking your own meals at home; but how do you choose the right foods when dining out? These guidelines were designed to help you eat right away from home.

- Avoid all fried and charcoal-grilled foods. This includes French fries, fried onions, and flame-cooked burgers and steaks. Fried food has cooked grease and oil in it, which contain trans-fatty acids. Trans-fatty acids will cause your psoriasis to break out or get worse. Charcoal-broiled meats have high levels of toxic compounds, which will contribute significantly to free-radical formation and oxidative stress.

- Use only *real* butter on your bread and other foods. Do not use margarine. Margarine and hydrogenated oils have trans-fatty acids. If you ask the waiter for butter, and you receive a plastic cup full of something soft and yellow, ask if it is real butter, or if it is just margarine. Don't use it if it is margarine or one of those hydrogenated oils.

- Stay away from pepper and its relatives, like cinnamon. Don't pepper your food, and don't order peppered food, such as "blackened" chicken, steak, or fish. Pepper taxes the liver. Lemon-pepper fish is also a "no-no." Ask to have yours prepared without the lemon pepper seasoning.

- Don't eat grapefruit or drink its juice. Don't eat foods containing turmeric; red chili pepper, which is in foods such as hot chili, many Mexican foods, or hot spicy Buffalo wings; or foods containing cloves or clove oil. All of these foods and spices inhibit the first phase of your liver's detoxification process. Smokers, however may benefit from eating turmeric.

- Order entrees with steamed broccoli; vitamin B-rich foods, such as whole-grain breads; and vitamin C-rich foods, such as red and green pepper.

- Eat high sulfur content foods, including those cooked with garlic, legumes, onions, and eggs. These will help protect your liver from damage and improve your liver function.

- Eat foods containing water-soluble fibers such as pears and apples.

- Stay away from vinegar. Order your salads without dressing. Try another topping, such as cheese, instead. Pickles are full of vinegar, so order your sandwiches and other foods minus the pickles. Also, don't order foods covered with vinegar-laden sauces, such as mayonnaise, ketchup, Worcestershire sauce, and other condiments.

- Order baked, broiled, or oven-grilled chicken, turkey, or fish more often than you order beef. Don't eat fatty meats, such as sausage and bacon for breakfast.

- Stay away from lemons, including lemon in your tea, lemonade, and lemon on your fish. The citric acid in lemons can increase oxygen free radicals and decrease levels of antioxidants in the body.

- Don't eat in noisy places, such as sports bars. Noise creates stress and will upset your digestion. You already have a problem with protein digestion—don't make it worse. I have found TGI Fridays and Applebee's to be very noisy at dinnertime. Places with large bar areas get rather noisy on Friday and Saturday nights. In addition, most of the menu selections at bars and grills are generally fried.

- Good places to eat out include restaurants with salad/ food bars. This gives you a chance to get your raw fruits and veggies with your meal. Cafeteria-style establishments are also good because of the quality of foods (including baked, broiled, or griddle-grilled meats) and types of foods (good selections of raw and cooked vegetables) available.

- Order foods and drinks that contain *no* alcohol. This includes main dishes and desserts. If you're not sure about whether or not something on the menu contains alcohol, ask your waiter or waitress. If the dish does contain alcohol, but you really like it, ask the cook to prepare it without the alcoholic beverage.

- Remember your allergies when ordering. Don't order something that will make you sick or break out in a rash later.

- If you crave steak, order one that is baked, such as prime rib, not char-grilled, like T-bone or ribeye. Ask how the steaks are cooked. Get yours baked or broiled.

- Always eat some type of protein with your other foods. Never eat only carbohydrates.

that help your body overcome the negative effects of medications, foods that reduce your inflammation, and foods that heal your bowels, glands, and liver. Keep reading to find out exactly what you can eat to fight your psoriasis.

As you follow these guidelines for your diet, you will also boost your immune system and decrease your risk of heart disease, cancer, stroke, and diabetes. You'll also learn key information, such as what foods are essential for you, which foods may help to prevent psoriasis symptoms, and how certain medications affect your need for nutrients.

Eat Foods Rich in Antioxidants

Antioxidants fight harmful molecules known as free radicals. There is a special unstable form of oxygen called singlet oxygen, which is created in your body during normal bodily reactions. This singlet oxygen is a free radical. It causes a lot of damage while it tries to become stable by stealing electrons from other molecules in your body. Antioxidants stop this damage by stabilizing the singlet oxygen.

Some antioxidants are vitamin A, vitamin C, vitamin E, and the mineral selenium. Your best defense against free-radical damage is to get your antioxidants from whole foods, but the soil in which the fruits and vegetables you eat were grown greatly influences the amount of vitamins and minerals they contain, so you'll probably still need to take supplements to help treat and prevent your psoriasis. See Chapter 5 for more information about antioxidant supplements.

Buy organically grown produce when you can to reduce your exposure to pesticide residues. Thoroughly wash your fruits and vegetables to remove surface pesticide residues, waxes, fungicides, and fertilizers.

Don't eat fruits or drink fruit juices by themselves as a meal without eating some protein if you have a low-blood-sugar problem. The sugars in the fruit or juice will cause your blood sugar levels to rise quickly and produce a large release of insulin. This will make it hard for you to get your blood sugar back under control. Be sure to eat some form of protein whenever you eat something with sugar if you have hypoglycemia.

Vitamin-A- and Carotenoid-Rich Foods

Carotenoids are precursors to vitamin A. Your body converts them into vitamin A. They also have their own beneficial properties. You'll get your vitamin A and carotenoids in yellow-orange fruits and vegetables, including apricots, sweet potatoes, pumpkins, carrots, cantaloupe and other melons, mangoes, papayas, peaches, and winter squash. You can also get it by eating dark green leafy vegetables, including broccoli, spinach, collard greens, and parsley. Some animal foods, such as liver, turkey, and milk, have vitamin A.

Vitamin-C-Rich Foods

You'll find vitamin C in fresh fruits, such as cantaloupes, grapefruit, papayas, kiwis, mangoes, raspberries, pineapples, bananas, strawberries, and tomatoes, and fresh vegetables, such as Brussels sprouts, collard greens, cabbage, asparagus, broccoli, potatoes, and red peppers. Vitamin C is heat-sensitive, and is destroyed in the cooking process, so cook these foods as little as possible—steam or microwave fruits and vegetables for as short a time as possible. Cut them after cooking, not before cooking, to keep most of the vitamin C inside.

Vitamin-E-Rich Foods

You can get vitamin E by eating sunflower and safflower oils, sunflower seeds, wheat germ, nuts, avocados, peaches, whole-grain breads and cereals, spinach, broccoli, asparagus, dried prunes, and peanut butter.

Selenium-Rich Foods

You can get your selenium by eating swordfish, salmon, tuna, cracked wheat bread, sunflower seeds, oysters, and shrimp.

Eat fresh vegetables, fresh fruit, whole grains (brown rice, wheat, oats, etc.), beans, and raw seeds and nuts to get your antioxidants. Be sure to include those foods rich in vitamins A, C, and E every day. Eat at least one of the selenium-rich foods every week. You can also take a supplement to get your vitamins A, C, and E, and selenium. See Chapter 5 to find out how much you should take.

Eat Foods Rich in Bioflavonoids

Bioflavonoids are substances found in almost all plant foods. You need them for healthy capillary walls and to be able to use vitamin C. They help your skin by reinforcing collagen, by preventing free-radical damage, by slowing inflammation reactions, and by hastening healing. Fresh fruits (particularly berries and fruits with pits), fresh vegetables (including onions), seeds, whole grains, and green tea have bioflavonoids.

Eat Foods That Offset the Negative Effects of Medications

You may be suffering from nutrient deficiencies caused by the prescription and over-the-counter medicines you have taken. Medications can affect the way your body uses certain vitamins and minerals. For example, high doses of aspirin can make you absorb less vitamin C. It will also make you lose iron and folic acid due to the bleeding it can cause in your stomach and intestines. Indocin (indomethacin) also causes you to lose iron and vitamin C. Foods that will offset the negative effects of these medications include foods containing vitamin C, iron, folic acid, and phosphorus. See page 116 for foods rich in vitamin C. Foods rich in the rest of these nutrients are discussed below.

If you take aspirin, eat more foods that have lots of vitamin C, iron, and folic acid every day. If you take indomethacin, eat foods that have lots of iron each day and keep your intake of sodium as low as you can.

Corticosteroids make you excrete zinc, potassium, and vitamin C. To compensate, you need to decrease your salt intake and eat more foods containing zinc, potassium, and vitamin C. Eat low-fat, low-calorie foods to offset your increased appetite.

Some people take antacids containing aluminum or magnesium hydroxide to counteract the stomach and intestinal problems caused by NSAIDs. These antacids can prevent your body from absorbing enough phosphorus into the bloodstream. You can counteract this effect by eating foods rich in phosphorus.

Iron-Rich Foods

Lean red meat, cooked dried beans and peas, dark leafy vegetables, fish, poultry, prunes and prune juice, oysters, and whole-grain breads and cereals are rich in iron.

Folic-Acid-Rich Foods

Eat dark green, leafy vegetables, avocados, beets, and broccoli, and drink orange juice to get more folic acid in your diet.

Phosphorus-Rich Foods

Eat meat, fish, poultry, eggs, nonfat milk, low-fat yogurt, soybeans, whole-wheat breads, cooked broccoli, bananas, cooked carrots, nuts, seeds, and peanut butter to get more phosphorus in your diet.

Zinc-Rich Foods

Oysters, lean meat, poultry, fish, whole-grain breads and cereals, and pumpkin seeds are rich in zinc.

Potassium-Rich Foods

Eat lean meats, potatoes, avocados, bananas, apricots, dried fruits, cooked dried beans, and peas, and drink orange juice to obtain potassium in your diet.

You may sometimes need medications prescribed for you, but they can be a threat to your health by depleting you of nutrients. Find out if your current medicines interfere with your absorption or use of any nutrients. You need to take in more of these nutrients either as supplements or in your food to compensate. After you get started on the Psoriasis Cure Program, you may find you won't need these medicines that rob your body of nutrients anymore.

Eat Foods That Help Reduce Inflammation and Plaques on Your Skin

Fatty acids can alter your body's inflammation response for the better or for the worse. Arachidonic acid is the fatty acid in the animal products and saturated fats you eat. It is the precursor to the bad type of prostaglandin—the kind that can harden your arteries, give you heart disease and strokes, and make your skin inflamed. The enzyme cyclooxygenase normally degrades arachidonic acid. Avoid aspirin because it inhibits cyclooxygenase. Egg yolks, poultry, dairy products, and meat all contain arachidonic acid. Does this mean you can't eat the foods you love? No, it just means you need to think about what you eat so you will minimize the impact of your food on your skin.

The best way to fight inflammation in your skin naturally is to consume lots of omega-3 and omega-6 fatty acids. Mackerel, anchovies, herring, salmon, sardines, lake trout, Atlantic sturgeon, and tuna contain eicosapentaenoic acid (EPA), the most beneficial of the omega-3 fatty acids. You need to eat two to five meals with one of these types of fish every week or to take a supplement containing omega-3 and omega-6 fatty acids every day. After you get your psoriasis under control so your skin shows no outward signs (no redness, no inflammation, no scales), you can cut back on eating these types of fish to once a week or once a month. You are the best judge of what works best for you. Don't fry your fish. That will destroy the omega-3 fatty acids.

Corn, soybean, sunflower, safflower, and flaxseed oils contain linoleic acid. This fatty acid reduces your inflammatory response. Make sure to consume one tablespoon of at least one of these oils every day.

You may want to get your omega-3 fatty acids from a nutritional supplement instead of from eating fish. That's OK, but you need to know that if you take too much, you can harm your blood's ability to clot. Also, fish oil has lots of vitamins A and D, and taking too much can lead to a toxic overdose of these vitamins. See Chapter 5 for more information about supplemental essential fatty acids.

Onion, garlic, and foods containing vitamin E will also help reduce inflammation by getting rid of the extra arachidonic acid in the psoriasis-afflicted areas of your skin.

Eat Foods That Heal Your Gastrointestinal System and Support Your Immune System

Once you get your bowels, glands, immune system, and liver more healthy, you'll see the results as clear, psoriasis-free skin. Use the Food Guide Pyramid below to help you select the foods you eat and

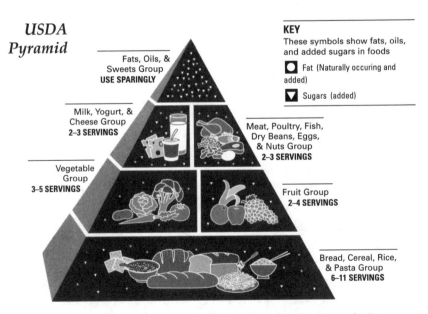

Source: U.S. Department of Agriculture and the U.S. Department of Health and Human Services.

to help you decide how much of each to have. Take the supplements you need. Focus on natural (with no preservatives), whole (uncooked, unprocessed) foods rich in the nutrients you need for your condition. Run away from saturated fats and hydrogenated oils like you would run from a snake coiled to strike. Don't eat heavily marbled or fatty meats. Also, don't eat the dark meat or skin of poultry. Don't eat visible fat. Don't ever skip a meal. Drink lots of water (eight to ten glasses a day) to help your body flush out toxic waste products. Don't go on fad diets. Make changes gradually, and keep this method of eating up until it becomes a habit.

Eating for Healthy Bowels, Stomach, and Pancreas

To get the most benefit from the food you eat, you have to digest, absorb, and eliminate it properly. You can eat wonderfully healthy foods, but it will be wasted if your body can't use it. A lack of acid in your stomach can inhibit digestion. (See "Signs and Symptoms of Low Stomach Acid" on page 122.) You can take enzyme supplements to help reduce this problem. Psoriasis sufferers should not take supplemental hydrochloric acid for problems with diminished hydrochloric acid secretion because this may worsen your psoriasis.

Psoriasis is a disease associated with low stomach acid. Obesity; cigarette smoking; eating chocolate and fried foods; and drinking carbonated beverages, alcohol, and coffee can give you heartburn by causing the contents of your stomach to flow upward back into the esophagus. Eliminate from your diet those foods and drinks that cause heartburn in your body.

You should have a bowel movement every twelve to fourteen hours. You need to eat plenty of fruits, vegetables, whole grains, beans, nuts, and seeds to ensure this. This type of diet will increase the frequency and quantity of your bowel movements; decrease the time between eating food and eliminating the wastes; decrease your absorption of toxins from the stool; and help prevent colon disorders, such as constipation, colon cancer, diverticulitis, hemorrhoids, and irritable bowel syndrome. Reduce the amount of sugar in your diet—sugar will cause such problems in your bowels as diarrhea and yeast infections. Drink plenty of water. Eat yogurt to maintain health-promoting microflora in your gastrointestinal system.

The color of your feces can indicate various conditions in your

Signs and Symptoms of Low Stomach Acid

Hydrochloric acid in the stomach is necessary for proper digestion, as well as the overall health of the body. The presence of any of the symptoms listed below may indicate a problem with diminished hydrochloric acid production. If you have a problem with low stomach acid, you should supplement your diet with digestive enzymes to aid the digestive process. If your symptoms do not go away, see your doctor.

- Feeling of uncomfortable fullness after eating.
- Acne.
- Bloating, belching, burning, and flatulence immediately after meals.
- Chronic *Candida* infections.
- Dilated blood vessels in the cheeks and nose.
- Indigestion, diarrhea, or constipation.
- Iron deficiency.
- Itching around the rectum.
- Multiple food allergies.
- Nausea after taking supplements.
- Undigested food in the stool.
- Upper-digestive-tract gassiness.
- Weak, peeling, and cracked fingernails.

gastrointestinal tract. If your feces are yellow to green, it may indicate that all of the beneficial bacteria in your lower gastrointestinal tract have been killed by antibiotics. Black stools can indicate upper-gastrointestinal-tract bleeding. Tan or gray greasy stools can indicate blockage of the common bile duct, severe pancreatic insufficiency, and fat malabsorption. Red stools may indicate possible lower gastrointestinal tract bleeding. Blood mixed in your stool may indicate bleeding in your colon, caused by anything from hemorrhoids to colon cancer. Mucus or pus can indicate irritable bowel syndrome or intestinal-wall inflammation caused by infection, diverticulitis, or other intestinal abscess.

Pancreatic enzymes are needed for proper protein digestion. Incomplete digestion of protein can lead to food allergies. If your pancreas isn't making enough enzymes, you may have abdominal bloating and discomfort, gas, and indigestion, and you may pass undigested food in your stool. You can take pancreatic enzymes as a supplement or get protein-digesting enzymes from eating pineapple (bromelain) and papaya (papain).

Microorganisms in your bowels can produce toxic substances. Vitamin A and goldenseal will inhibit enzymes that harmful bacteria in your bowels need to turn amino acids into toxic compounds. Eat foods containing vitamin A. Your diet should be rich in water-soluble fiber to reduce the absorption of toxic substances in your bowels. You can get this fiber in vegetables, the guar gum found in some powdered fiber supplements, the pectin found in apples, and oat bran. Fiber can bind to the toxins in your gut and help your body excrete them.

Eating for Healthy Glands and Immune Function Support

Your thymus gland is an important part of your immune system. The health of your thymus will greatly determine the health of your immune system. You must take in vitamin A, carotenoids, vitamin C, vitamin E, the B vitamins, iron, zinc, and selenium every day to support your immune system and keep your thymus gland from shrinking. See pages 116 through 117 for foods rich in these nutrients. Nutrient deficiency has been said to be the most common cause of immune system problems.

Reduce the amount of sugar in your diet. A high sugar intake will lead to lowered white blood cell activity. As little as 100 grams of sugar, such as glucose, fructose, sucrose, or honey can reduce your white blood cells' ability to destroy foreign particles and microorganisms. The negative effects of consuming sugar can last over five hours. As you eat more sugar, your white-blood-cell function lowers. So, the more sugar you eat, the more you hurt your immune system. Simple sugars, such as fruit juice, can impair your immune function, especially if you have an infection. Stay away from sugar if you want to boost your immune system while you have an infection. Read labels on the foods you eat. Some terms for added sugar include sucrose, glucose, maltose, lactose, fructose, corn syrup, or white grape juice concentrate.

Avoid alcohol, because it will also inhibit white-blood-cell activity. And be sure to eat some protein every day. Your body's immune system can't function properly without protein.

Eating for a Healthy Liver

The liver is a vital organ in the detoxification process. Your body eliminates toxins by neutralizing or excreting them. If not eliminated, these toxins will build up in your body's tissues causing harm.

Detoxification in the liver occurs in two phases. In Phase I of detoxification, toxins are chemically modified so that they are more easily detoxified by the enzymes sent to metabolize and eliminate them in Phase II. While Phase I is a necessary process in the elimination of toxins from the body, it can cause problems. Every time a toxin is metabolized in Phase I, harmful free radicals are produced. If the body does not have enough antioxidants to fight them, the free radicals will cause damage in the body. Also, after toxins are metabolized in Phase I, they are even more toxic than they were originally. If not eliminated from the body by the Phase II enzymes immediately, these toxins will cause great harm to the body. For these reasons, it is essential that the rates of Phases I and II are balanced.

A healthy liver is very important in keeping psoriasis symptoms at bay. You must eat healthfully in order to keep your liver healthy. Avoid saturated fats, refined sugar, and alcohol. Eat foods that help with Phase I and Phase II detoxification, including those with high sulfur content, such as garlic, legumes, onions, and eggs; those with water-soluble fiber, such as pears, oat bran, and apples; and cabbage-family vegetables, such as broccoli, Brussels sprouts, and cabbage. Beets, carrots, and dandelion greens will also help.

There are several drugs that will activate the first phase of detoxification. These include alcohol, nicotine in cigarette smoke, phenobarbital, sulfonamides, and steroids. If you take any of these drugs, your Phase I detoxification system will be more active than the Phase II system. You will need to offset these negative effects by taking in more nutrients to help heal your liver and stimulate Phase II.

Some foods also will stimulate the first phase of detoxification. These include charcoal-broiled meats (due to toxic compounds such as the carcinogen benzopyrene created by the contact of the flame with animal fat), oranges, and tangerines. Excessive consumption of protein can also stimulate this phase. Some herbs and spices, caraway seeds, dill seeds, and pepper will also cause your liver to work overtime. Avoid these.

Exposure to some environmental toxins will also cause your liver to work harder to protect you. These include carbon tetrachloride, exhaust fumes, paint fumes, dioxin, and pesticides. Avoid these if you can, and take more liver-helping nutrients if you are exposed.

There are several foods, drinks, and chemicals that will inhibit Phase I detoxification in your liver. You need to avoid these because they will make toxins more damaging to you—they will stay in your body longer before being removed by your liver. Drugs that inhibit Phase I detoxification include benzodiazepines (Halcion, Centrax, Librium, Valium, etc.), antihistamines, cimetidine and other stomach-acid secretion blocking drugs, ketoconazole, and sulfaphenazole. Foods that inhibit Phase I detoxification include grapefruit juice, the spice turmeric, red chili peppers (due to a component called capsaicin), and clove oil (due to a component called eugenol).

Certain foods, such as broccoli, cabbage, and Brussels sprouts stimulate both Phase I and Phase II detoxification. This is the ideal situation.

To help your liver in the detoxification process, eat glutathione-rich foods, such as fresh fruits and vegetables and cooked fish and meat. Asparagus, avocado, and walnuts are particularly rich in glutathione. Vitamin C (1,000 to 3,000 milligrams per day in divided doses) will increase your glutathione levels by helping your body make it.

Eat foods rich in the B vitamins choline, such as animal products, lecithin, soybeans, and whole-grain cereals; folic acid, such as green leafy vegetables; thiamine (vitamin B_2), such as beans, brown rice, and whole grains; pantothenic acid (vitamin B_5), such as beef, eggs, and brewer's yeast; vitamin B_6, such as whole grains, legumes, and animal products; and vitamin B_{12}, like brewer's yeast, eggs, dairy products, and seafood; and foods rich in vitamin C to help the liver in the detoxification process. The liver also uses several amino acids in the detoxification process. Make sure you are eating enough protein-rich foods to ensure the proper functioning of the liver.

The liver also uses sulfur in the detoxification process. Eat plenty of sulfur-containing foods, such as red peppers, garlic, onions, broccoli, and Brussels sprouts.

Some people recommend fasting as a method of detoxification. I personally would not suggest this to you because of two potentially dangerous problems. First, if you have hypoglycemia, your blood sugar levels could drop so low you could go into a coma. Second, if you have been exposed to fat-soluble toxins, such as pesticides, these will get into your bloodstream during a fast and could reach toxic levels in your body.

Aging will decrease the flow of blood through your liver. You can counteract this effect by being more physically active to increase your circulation and by eating only healthy foods. The elderly often have toxic reactions to drugs because they can't eliminate the drugs fast enough, causing them to build up in their bodies.

Help your bowels, stomach, and pancreas work to help you by eating foods containing vitamin A and by eating yogurt. If you don't have enough acid in your stomach, either eat enzyme-containing foods or take enzyme supplements. Help your glands and immune system by eating foods containing vitamin A, carotenes, vitamin C, vitamin E, the B vitamins, iron, zinc, and selenium every day. Also, reduce your sugar intake.

Help your liver get rid of the toxins in your blood by eating cabbage-family foods, vitamin B-rich foods, vitamin C-rich foods, high-sulfur content foods, and water-soluble fiber foods. Also, take a high-potency multiple-vitamin-and-mineral supplement and antioxidant vitamins, such as vitamins C and E.

PLAN YOUR MENU

You can easily eat well enough to prevent nutrient-deficiency dis-eases, such as beriberi or scurvy. A deficiency in any nutrient can leave your body weak and susceptible to disease. Your body needs lots of nutrients, including protein, carbohydrates, fats, fiber, vita-mins, and minerals, to keep everything working properly. You get these in different amounts and combinations in the foods you eat. If you eat the same foods all the time, you will be shortchanging your-self and depriving your body of nutrients it needs. Supercharge your health by enjoying a variety of foods.

This therapeutic diet will help you control some of your psoria-sis symptoms. Remember, variety is the spice of life, so pick differ-ent kinds of fruits, vegetables, and whole grains for each meal. You'll get bored eating the same things each time, and you can get food allergy reactions eating that way. Avoid eating the wrong foods.

You *must* eat breakfast every day. Never, ever skip breakfast. Never eat anything too sugary, like a donut, for breakfast. Eat some whole-grain cereals, muffins, or breads with fresh fruit or fruit juice. Include some form of protein (meat, eggs, seeds, or beans) with your breakfast. Have some more protein, such as beans or meat, and a vegetable, along with some whole-grain bread for lunch. Have something from each food group for dinner. Don't eat too many animal products. Eat fish, skinless poultry, and lean cuts of meat, instead of fat-laden meats.

There are lots of excellent cookbooks that will provide you with terrific recipes you can use to meet these dietary guidelines. As you alter your diet, make sure to keep a record of the recipes you like the most. See the inset on page 113 for tips that will help you when eating out. Remember that you need more protein to keep your psoriasis at bay than most nutritionists will recommend. Make protein compose at least 40 percent of every meal.

You now know the main elements of a psoriasis-relieving diet. You are now armed with information about what you need to eat to boost your immune system, to help heal your liver, glands, and bowels, and to reduce inflammation. Think of food as your medicine.

Beat Stress Before It Beats You

You need to know how to recognize and handle stress in your life to keep your psoriasis under control. Your body sends out floods of hormones in response to stress. These hormones can make your inflammation and scales worse and make you irritable and tired. You can't get rid of all your stress, but you can alter the way in which you respond to stress. The stress doesn't determine your body's response—your reaction to stress determines the response. Many things can cause a stress response in your body—a cold draft, driving in heavy traffic, being late for an important meeting, disease, injury, or joy. Stress is the spice of life because any emotion or activity will cause it. Some types of stress that one person may find invigorating will make another person sick. You must prepare your body to take the stresses of your life.

Physical signs of stress include insomnia, depression, fatigue, headache, upset stomach, digestive disturbances, and irritability. Have you ever experienced any of these? Treat your stress or teach yourself how to handle it instead of just treating the symptoms. Keep reading to discover how you can beat stress before it beats you.

WHAT IS STRESS?

Stress can be any type of disturbance, such as heat or cold, toxins from your environment or from microorganisms, strong emotional reactions, or physical trauma. These disturbances trigger biological changes in your body that produce the stress response. Sometimes this stress response is very mild and you don't notice it. When your stress is extreme or unusual or lasts too long, your body's response to stress will start causing quite a bit of harm to you.

YOUR BODY'S RESPONSE TO STRESS

Imagine you are taking a pleasant walk on a beautiful summer day through a wooded nature trail. Your enjoyment is cut rather short when you hear a funny rattling sound. You look around to see the source of the sound. At your feet, just a few feet away, is a rattlesnake ready to strike. How do you feel? This feeling is caused by adrenaline surging through your body. Your adrenal glands release adrenaline to give your body the extra energy you need to escape from danger, such as the rattlesnake. The problem with adrenaline is that it also makes you feel nervous and anxious when you are stressed.

If you are under prolonged stress, your heart, blood vessels, adrenal glands, and immune system will be harmed. Stress makes your adrenal glands release adrenaline and corticosteroids. These hormones inhibit your ability to form white blood cells and make your thymus gland shrink. This will make you more susceptible to infections, cancer, and other illnesses.

Adrenaline works on your nervous and immune systems. Everything in your body is affected by it. It is often called the "fight-or-flight" hormone, because it causes changes in your body that allow you to protect yourself. When you are scared or feel you are in danger, adrenaline is released. This takes energy away from your digestion so you can use that energy to run, fight, or protect yourself from the danger.

If you have too much adrenaline in your bloodstream, you will be tense and can't sit still. You will not be able to concentrate and will become agitated. Anything will make you aggressive or angry. Your body responds to stress in three phases—alarm, resistance, and exhaustion.

Your adrenal glands regulate and control these phases. The first thing your body does when you are stressed is to mobilize your body's resources for immediate physical activity so you can either fight or flee from the danger. Your adrenal glands can't tell the difference between real danger and an annoyance. They can't think, they just respond.

Alarm

In the alarm phase, your adrenal glands release adrenaline. The released adrenaline takes blood away from your skin and internal organs to allow more blood to go to the muscles to prepare you to fight or flee. Your breathing rate increases, your blood pressure rises, and you sweat more. The release of adrenaline also causes your digestive system to slow down and your blood-sugar levels to dramatically increase to prepare you to defend yourself.

Resistance

In the resistance phase, your adrenal cortex keeps your blood pressure elevated by secreting cortisol and other corticosteroids. Your body needs these changes to deal with danger, meet a crisis, or perform a strenuous task, but this overuse of your adrenal glands can lead to the third stage of the stress response—exhaustion.

Exhaustion

When your body has to continually fight physical or emotional stress, your adrenal glands will do the same thing that you do when you work very hard and get too tired—quit working and take a rest. If you get to the point of exhaustion, certain organs may stop working efficiently, or in the worst-case scenario, stop working altogether. When the cells of your body lose too much potassium, or your adrenal steroid hormones are depleted, they will not work as well and will eventually die. You will become hypoglycemic when your adrenal steroid hormones become depleted and your cells don't get enough glucose and other nutrients.

WHAT IS THE LINK BETWEEN STRESS AND PSORIASIS?

Stress makes your psoriasis worse by depleting vitamins and minerals that are essential to your health. This can lead to inflammation and dry skin. Stress also weakens your digestive system by reducing the amount of digestive enzymes you make. Fewer digestive enzymes means you don't digest your food very well, and toxins can build up. You've already learned that toxins in your stomach and intestines can result in the formation of psoriasis scales because of an imbalance in those substances that regulate skin cell growth and maturation.

WHO IS AT RISK FOR BECOMING OVERSTRESSED?

Doctors use a rating scale to determine the role stress plays in your health problems. This rating scale is called the Social Readjustment Rating Scale, developed by Holmes and Rahe. It is used to predict the likelihood of your getting a serious disease from your body's response to your stress. Quite a few life-change events are rated according to how much they can cause disease. Some events viewed as positive, such as outstanding personal acheivement, also are rated because they cause stress. If you are under a great deal of stress right now, or have endured a good bit of stress over the past few months or longer, your adrenal glands have probably suffered and need help.

Life events have a strong effect on your stress level, but not everyone reacts to a life event in the same way. Have you had any of the following stressful events in your life? This will give you a rough idea of how much stress you are dealing with.

- Death of a spouse.

- Divorce.

- Death of a close family member.

- Personal injury or illness.

- Marriage.

- Change in financial status.

- Change to a different line of work.

- Son or daughter leaving home.

- Beginning or ending school.

- Being fired at work.

- Pressure at work.

- Retirement.

- Pregnancy.

- Gain of a new family member.

- Death of a close friend.

- Changes in living conditions.

HOW CAN YOU BEAT STRESS?

You must focus on five key areas to deal effectively with your stress. These key areas are:

- Mental calming and attitude-uplifting techniques.

- Lifestyle changes—managing time and relationships.

- Exercise.

- Healthy diet.

- Whole body and adrenal gland support.

Calming and Uplifting Techniques

You must learn how to calm your mind and body so you can relieve stress and get rid of your psoriasis. Stress will melt away like ice on a summer day when your mind and body are calm. An easy way to quiet your body and mind is to use relaxation exercises. You can use relaxation exercises to produce the relaxation response—the opposite response of the stress response—in your body. This is much deeper relaxation than you can get by watching television or reading a book.

Your stress response is controlled by the sympathetic nervous system, which focuses on protecting you from immediate danger. Your relaxation response is controlled by your parasympathetic nervous system, which focuses on repairing, restoring, and maintaining your body. You can use a variety of techniques to achieve the relaxation response. The most common ones are progressive relaxation, imagery, massage therapy, and yoga. You pick the best technique for you. Set aside five to ten minutes each day to perform one of these techniques.

Before you try any of these techniques, you need to learn how to breathe. Yes, I said breathe. But I already know how to breathe, you say. I'm doing it now. Yes, but are you breathing with your diaphragm? Deep relaxation techniques require breathing with your diaphragm. You can activate the relaxation centers in your brain by using your diaphragm to breathe. Here's how you need to breathe when you really want and need to relax:

1. Sit or lie down in a quiet, comfortable place where you won't be disturbed. Wear comfortable, nonbinding clothes.

2. Put one hand on your stomach just above your navel. Put the other hand on your chest.

3. Close your mouth. Breathe in through your nose and breathe out through your mouth.

4. Think about your breathing. Forget about everything else. Pay attention to which hand is going up and which hand is going down with every breath you take.

5. Empty your lungs by breathing out gently.

6. Breathe in to a count of four, while keeping your chest and shoulders still and expanding your abdomen.

7. Think of the air entering you as warmth flowing all over your body, your hands, your feet, your head, your legs, your arms.

8. Breathe out to a count of four.

9. Let your mind see tension and stress leave your body.

10. Keep doing this until you feel very relaxed.

Progressive relaxation involves forcefully contracting and then relaxing your muscles to achieve relaxation. Start with your head, then go down to your feet, slowly contracting and then relaxing all of your muscles. There are some wonderful cassette tapes available in book and music stores that will help you do this.

Aromatherapy will also help melt away stress at the end of your day and ease the transition between work and home. Put a drop or two of relaxing clary sage and lavender essential oils on a tissue or napkin and place it on the dashboard of your car. Then let it heat up in the sun. The heat will release the fragrant oils and help you calm down.

The use of imagery can help you become more relaxed. Close your eyes, and see yourself as a feather floating in the air. Relax as you drift down to the ground. As you leave your job at the end of the day, let your stress run out your feet as a liquid with each step, so you leave colored footprints on the ground representing your stress. Let the footprints fade as you walk further from your job, and let the stress fade as the footprints fade.

Massage can relieve the tense neck and shoulder muscles resulting from stress. Reflexology is a good way to relax and ward off stress. It is a type of massage therapy in which it is believed that reflex areas on the feet correspond to every part of the body. It is especially useful for stimulating deep relaxation. Make sure your therapist pays special attention to the areas that correspond to the diaphragm; the spine; and the pituitary, parathyroid, thyroid, and adrenal glands.

Listen to some relaxing music while lying comfortably on a couch or on the floor. Bend your knees slightly and put a rounded folded towel under your neck to support it. Allow the music to wash over you and rinse away the stress of your day. Concentrate on your breathing.

Yoga is a system of health that incorporates lifestyle changes, detoxification methods, breathing control, meditation, and yogic postures. It is a stress-buster you can practice anywhere, anytime you feel stressed. There are several yoga institutes across the country and books about yoga that can provide you with information for practicing it. Consult your local health-food store for information about these sources of information. Try different yoga poses every day to teach your mind and body to relax and give you a quick mental vacation when you need one.

Lifestyle Changes

Your level of stress is directly tied to your lifestyle. The two biggest concerns are time management and relationships.

Manage Your Time

Do you ever feel rushed, like you don't have enough time? This is a big stressor. Here are a few ways you can manage your time to feel less stressed.

- Take some time every day, at the same time every day, to figure out what you have to do for that day or the next day. Make a written list. Now, decide which things on that list are most important. Rank them in order of priority. Work on getting the most important things done first. If you don't get the less important things done by the end of the day, don't worry about it. Focus your efforts on getting the most important things done.

- Become organized and plan your day. Unfortunately, you'll always have someone or something interrupt you and place unplanned demands on your time, but for the most part, you can create a plan for your day in accordance with your written list of important things to do. Don't spend your life "putting out fires." If you let them, immediate demands will control your life.

- You can't do everything yourself, and you will become very stressed if you try, so get others to help you when possible. Train other people to do what needs to be done, then depend on them.

- Get the tough stuff out of the way first. Do the most important things on your list first while you have enough energy to complete them.

- Make your meetings as short as possible so they don't eat up your time. Have meetings scheduled so they have a natural end point, such as lunch time.

- Don't put things off. Give yourself a reasonable deadline to avoid becoming so stressed that you do a bad job or that you are too apprehensive to start at all.

- Don't try to do everything perfectly. You'll be so worried about getting everything just right, you may never start. Allow a reasonable amount of time to do your best, then go on to your other important tasks.

Manage Your Relationships

Effective communication is the key to reducing stress in your marital, family, and job-related interpersonal relationships. Learn how to communicate effectively so you can reduce conflicts in your interpersonal relationships and reduce stress. Some of the ways you can do this are:

- Learn how to be a good listener. Let other people talk. Don't interrupt. Remain interested and listen fully to what others are saying before thinking about how you will respond to what they are saying. Really try to understand the other person's point of view. Ask questions to get more information or to clear up anything you don't understand. Let the other person know you are listening and understanding by restating back to the other person what they said to you in your words. That will help you be better understood once you express your feelings.

- Don't talk until the people you want to communicate with are listening to you. You'll be wasting your time otherwise because they won't hear you.

- If someone interrupts you while you are talking, remain calm; don't start a shouting match. Be courteous. Let them speak, then point out that they are interrupting you.

- Make sure other people understood what you were trying to say by asking them to tell you what they heard. Sometimes, when you think you were crystal clear, the message was lost or confused before it reached the mind of the other person. If the other person didn't understand, say it another way until they do understand.

- Silence is also a form of communication. Don't let silence make you uncomfortable. Some people need some time, in silence, to collect their thoughts.

Exercise

Exercise causes stress on your body, but over time the body adapts. It helps you become stronger, function more efficiently, and be able to endure more stress. It is a critical part of your comprehensive stress management program. Want to get rid of that old tired feeling and depression? Regular exercise—something that isn't too strenuous that you enjoy doing—will drive away tension, depression, worry, and feelings of inadequacy. It will greatly improve your mood and your ability to handle anything life throws at you.

Healthy Diet

You can help your body handle stress better by eliminating or restricting the amount of caffeine you take in. This includes tea, coffee, chocolate, and other similar caffeinated drinks and foods. Some people are so affected by caffeine, they are even affected by the trace amounts of caffeine remaining in decaffeinated coffee. Caffeine can cause you to become depressed, nervous, and irritable and have headaches, heart palpitations, and insomnia.

You should also eliminate or restrict the amount of alcohol you drink. Alcohol is a toxin and will damage many parts of your body. It makes your adrenal glands pour out more hormones, interferes with your normal sleep patterns, and alters your brain chemistry. Do you think alcohol will help make you calm? It doesn't. Studies have shown that it significantly increases anxiety.

Quit eating refined carbohydrates. That means no more of those sugary donuts, pastries, cakes, or snacks. Sugar and white flour make your hypoglycemia problems worse. Many people who experience depression, anxiety, or other psychological conditions have hypoglycemia. Good therapy for depression or anxiety due to hypoglycemia is to simply eliminate refined carbohydrates.

Eat more foods with potassium and fewer foods with sodium. Remember that your cells will die if they lose too much potassium. Potassium supports your adrenal glands.

Plan your meals. Eat breakfast, lunch, and dinner in a calm way in a calm place. Eating in a noisy place will also cause you to become stressed.

Discover and control your food allergies. Anxiety, fatigue, muscle and joint aches, drowsiness, difficulty concentrating, and depression are key features of food allergies.

Think about the foods you have eaten over the past several days. How much of it was full of sugar, fat, and cholesterol? Your body can't become strong enough to fend off the effects of your stress if it doesn't get enough high-quality nutrition.

Whole Body and Adrenal Gland Support

You can help your whole body and support your adrenal glands by supplementing your diet with key nutrients, and using botanical medicines to help your adrenal glands.

Nutritional Supplements

Your adrenal glands need vitamin C, pantothenic acid, vitamin B_6, zinc, and magnesium to be healthy and make adrenal hormones. You can become deficient in these nutrients when you are stressed. You excrete more vitamin C in your urine when you are physically, chemically, or emotionally stressed. You are the best judge of how much you are stressed and how much extra vitamin C you may need. Pantothenic acid (vitamin B_5) supports your adrenal glands. You will become tired, will not be able to sleep, and will get headaches, nausea, and abdominal pains if you become deficient in this vitamin from stress. If you suffer from chronic stress or have used corticosteroids, supplement your diet with 100 to 500 milligrams of pantothenic acid every day. See Chapter 5 for guidelines on taking the proper supplements for eradicating your psoriasis and for overall health.

Botanical Medicines

Chinese ginseng (*Panax ginseng*) and Siberian ginseng (*Eleutherococcus senticosus*) help your adrenal glands and help you to resist stress. They increase the tone and function of your adrenal glands. They can restore your vitality, help you feel more energetic, help your mental and physical performance, counteract the negative effects of cortisone, help your liver work better, help your body resist the bad effects of stress better, and protect you from radiation damage. The best ginseng for you if you have been under a lot of stress, are recovering from a long illness, or have taken corticosteroids for a long time is Chinese ginseng. If your stress is moderate, Siberian ginseng is better.

Stress can make your psoriasis worse by causing your skin to become inflamed and scaly. It can also make you depressed, tired, and irritable. You can protect yourself against these effects by managing your stress with calming and uplifting techniques, managing your time, communicating better in your relationships, exercising, eating healthy, and supporting your body and adrenal glands with vitamins and botanical medicines.

Conclusion

Millions needlessly suffer with the symptoms of psoriasis daily, as well as with the adverse side effects of drugs used to treat the condition. However, as you have learned from reading this book, you can now safely and effectively prevent, treat, and even cure your psoriasis—all without using drugs or other dangerous methods!

You may have experienced unpleasant and even dangerous side effects from taking artificial prescription drugs. These effects on your body are called "contraindications" by pharmaceutical firms to lessen your repulsion to them and your fear of taking the drug. Look at the long list of scary things that can happen to you on the package insert of the medicine you are now taking.

Following the Psoriasis Cure Program, you can be happier, healthier, and less dependent on doctors; enjoy more energy; sleep better; get sick less frequently; and save tons of money that would have been spent on medical care. Finally, after enduring the frustration and embarrassment of psoriasis, feeling tired and listless all the time, and wondering how much worse your psoriasis is going to get, you can do something about it.

You have learned how such factors as allergies, stress, nutrient deficiencies, and poor detoxification of the body can trigger flares of your psoriasis. Now, put the Psoriasis Cure to work for you. Eliminate those foods from your diet and things in your life that cause your psoriasis symptoms. Supplement your diet with vitamin, mineral, essential-fatty-acid, and herbal supplements. Eat right, and exercise.

Traditional medicine approaches your psoriasis by attacking your pocketbook, and often offers you danger as well. The natural methods shown in *The Psoriasis Cure* offer an inexpensive, effective, and safe alternative. When used properly, the potential side effects are negligible or nonexistent. You'll strengthen your immune system, increase your energy level, and relieve your symptoms of psoriasis. This method works *with* your body, not against it. You won't have to suffer the damage you get from so many of the aggressive, artificial, and invasive methods of traditional medicine that fight your body.

Many people could benefit dramatically from this information if only they knew about it and how to take advantage of it. That's why *The Psoriasis Cure* was written. Follow the advice in *The Psoriasis Cure*, and you'll see truly astounding benefits to your health. It contains information and advice with the power to improve your health and well-being immediately. Seize this opportunity to find out for yourself how well it works.

It is possible to overcome the disfiguring and disabling effects of psoriasis with the Psoriasis Cure. It is a simple program—start today!

Endnotes

Chapter 3

[1] McKenna, K.E. and P.S. Stern. "Photosensitivity Associated With Combined UV-B and Calcipotriene Therapy." *Archives of Dermatology* 131 (1995):1305–1307.

[2] Cook, J.W., C.L. Hewett, and I. Hieger. "The isolation of cancer producing hydrocarbons from coal tar." *Journal of the American Chemical Society* 1933: 396–405.

[3] van Schooten, F.J. and R. Godschalk. "Coal tar therapy: is it carcinogenic?" *Drug Safety* 15 (6) (Dec 1996):374–377.

[4] Pion, I.A., K.L. Koenig, and H.W. Lim. "Is dermatologic usage of coal tar carcinogenic? A review of the literature." *Dermatological Surgery* 21 (Mar 1995):227–232.

[5] Carle, Paul, MD, et al. "Epstein-Barr Virus-Associated Lymphoproliferative Disease During Methotrexate Therapy for Psoriasis." *Archives of Dermatology* 133 (7) (July 1997): 805–938

[6] Smith, D. "Sulfasalazine: Arthritis Drug Increases CD4 Count?" *AIDS Treatment News* 218 (March 3, 1995).

[7] Grossman, R.M., et al. "Long-Term Safety of Cyclosporine in the Treatment of Psoriasis." *Archives of Dermatology* 132 (1996):623–629.

[8] Schütz, E, et al. "Azathioprine pharmacogenetics: the relationship between 6-thioguanine nucleotides and thiopurine methyl-

transferase in patients after heart and kidney transplantation."
European Journal of Clinical Chemistry and Clinical Biochemistry 34(3)
(Mar 1996):199–205

[9] Zackheim, H.S., et al. "6-Thioguanine treatment of psoriasis:
experience in 81 patients." *Journal of the American Academy of
Dermatology* 30(3) (Mar 1994):452–458.

[10] Buccheri, Katchen, Cohen, and Korter, *The Albert Einstein College
of Medicine (AECOM),* http://www.aecom.yu.edu

[11] DiGiovanna, J.J., et al. "Osteoporosis Is a Toxic Effect of Long-
Term Etretinate Therapy." *Archives of Dermatology* 131 (1995):
1263–1267.

[12] Department of Medicine, College of Medicine, King Saud
University, Riyadh, Saudi Arabia. *International Journal of
Dermatology,* 35(3) (March 1996):212–215.

[13] The European FK 506 Multicentre Psoriasis Study Group.
"Systemic Tacrolimus (FK 506) in Double-Blind Study." *Archives of
Dermatology* 132 (1996):419–423. Y

Chapter 5

[1] The World Health Organization

[2] M.D. Zanoli, "Psoriasis and Reiter's Disease," in *Principles and
Practice of Dermatology,* ed. W.M. Sams, Jr and P.J. Lynch, (New
York: Churchill Livingstone, 1990), pp. 307–323.

[3] N.B. Zlatkov, J.J. Ticholov, and A.L. Dourmishev, "Free Fatty
Acids in the Blood Serum of Psoriatics," *Acta Dermato-Venereologica
(stockh)* 64 (1984):22–25.

[4] S.B. Bittiner, et al, "A Double-Blind, Randomized, Placebo-
Controlled Trial of Fish Oil in Psoriasis," *Lancet* i (1988):378–380.

[5] F. Grimmunger, et al, "A Double-Blind, Randomized, Placebo-
Controlled Trial of N-3 Fatty Acid Based Lipid Infusion in Acute,
Extended Guttate Psoriasis," *Journal of Clinical Investigation* 71
(1993):634–643.

[6] P.D.L. Maurice, et al, "The Effects of Dietary Supplementation
with Fish Oil in Patients with Psoriasis," *British Journal of
Dermatology* 1117 (1987):599–606.

[7] S. Majewski, et al, "Decreased Levels of Vitamin A in Serum of Patients with Psoriasis," *Archives of Dermatological Research* 280 (1989):499–501.

[8] emery@sfsuvax1.sfsu.edu (Emery Dora). Psoriasis Research.

[9] M. Haddox, K. Frassir, and D. Russel, "Retinol Inhibition of Ornithine Decarboxylase Induction and G1 Progression in CHD Cells," *Cancer Research* 39 (1979):4930–4938.

[10].S. Kuwano and K. Yamauchi. "Effect of Berberine on Tyrosine Decarboxylase Activity of Streptococcus Faecalis," *Chemical & Pharmaceutical Bulletin* 8 (1960):491–496.

[11] P. Dowd and R. Heatley, "The Influence of Undernutrition on Immunity," *Clinical Science* 66 (1984):241–248.

[12] Dowd and Heatley, *Clinical Science,* 241–248.

[13] A. Bendick, "Vitamin C and Immune Responses," *Food and Technology* 41 (1987):112–114.

[14] B. Staberg, A. Oxholm, P. Klemp, and C. Christiansen. "Abnormal Vitamin D Metabolism in Patients with Psoriasis," *Acta Dermato-Venereologica* (*Stockh*) 67 (1987):65–68.

[15] M.M. Molokhia, and B. Portnoy. "Zinc and Copper in Dermatology," in *Zinc and Copper in Medicine,* ed. Zeymel, A., et. al. (Springfield, IL: Charles C. Thomas, 1980)

[16] K. Schmidt, et.al., "Determination of trace element concentrations in psoriatic and non-psoriatic scales with special attention to zinc," *Trace Element Analytical Chemistry in Medicine and Biology,* Vol. 1. (New York: Walter de Gruyter, 1980).

[17] E.M. McMillan and D. Rowe, "Plasma zinc in psoriasis. Relation to surface area involvement." *British Journal of Dermatology* 108 (1983):301.

[18] R.J. Ecker and A.L. Schroeder, "Acrodermatitis and acquired zinc deficiency," *Archives of Dermatology* 114 (1978): 937.

[19] Nutrition 21, "Selenium and Fat Metabolism," *Health Supplement News,* http://www.nutrition21.com (August 1, 1996).

[20] L. Juhlin, L. Bedquist, G. Echman, et al., "Blood Glutathione-Peroxide Levels in Skin Diseases: Effect of Selenium and Vitamin E Treatment," *Acta Dermato-Venereologica* (*Stock*) 62 (1982):211–214.

[21] L. Kiremidjian-Schumacher and G. Stotsky, "Selenium and Immune Responses," *Environmental Research* 42 (1987):277–303.

[22] P. Fratino, C. Pelfini, A. Jucci, and R. Bellazi, "Glucose and Insulin in Psoriasis: The Role of Obesity and Genetic History," *Panminerva Medica* 21 (1979):167.

[23] G. Weber and K. Galle, "The Liver, a Therapeutic Target in Dermatoses," *Die Medizinische Welt* 34 (1983):108–111.

[24] H.A. Salmi and S. Sarna, "Effect of Silymarin on Chemical, Functional, and Morphological Alteration of the Liver: A Double-Blind Controlled Study," *Scandinavian Journal of Gastroenterology* 17 (1981):417–421.

[25] C. Boari et al., "Occupational Toxic Liver Diseases: Therapeutic Effects of Silymarin," *Minerva Medica* 72 (1985):2679–2688.

[26] A. Klein et al., "The Effect of Nonviral Liver Damage on the T-Lymphocyte Helper/Suppressor Ratio," *Clinical Immunology and Immunopathology* 46 (1988):214–220.

[27] R. Bauer and H. Wagner, "Echinacea Species as Potential Immunostimulatory Drugs," *Econ Medicinal Plant Research* 5 (1991):253–321.

[28] M. Proctor, et. al., "Lowered Cutaneous and Urinary Levels of Polyamines with Clinical Improvement in Treated Psoriasis," *Archives of Dermatology* 115 (1979):945–949.

[29] J. Voorhees and E. Duell, "Imbalanced Cyclic AMP-Cyclic GMP Levels in Psoriasis," *Advances in Cyclic Nucleotide Research* 5 (1975):755–757.

[30] S. Robbins and R. Cotran, *Pathological Basis of Disease* (Philadelphia: W B Saunders, 1979), p. 449.

[31] G. Prasad and V.D. Sharma, "Efficacy of Garlic Treatment Against Experimental Candidiasis in Chicks," *British Veterinary Journal* 136 (1980):448–451.

[32] G. F. Kroker, "Chronic Candidiasis and Allergy," in *Food Allergy and Intolerance*, ed. J. Brostoff and S.J. Challacombe (Philadelphia: W. G. Saunders, 1987), p. 850–872.

[33] See Numbers 11:5 in the Bible.

Index

nutrient-rich, 115–117, 118–119
Free radicals, 64–65
    psoriasis and, 22

G
Gamma-linolenic acid (GLA), 24–25, 66, 67–68
Garlic oil, 87–88
Gastrointestinal system health, foods and, 120–123
Ginseng, 139–140
GLA. *See* Gamma-linolenic acid.
Glucagon, 17
Glutathione, 84
Glutathione peroxidase, 23
Goals, setting positive, 106–109
Goeckerman treatment, the, 33
Goldenseal, 84–85
Greer's Goo, 30
Guttate psoriasis, 10

H
Halcinonide, 29
Halobetasol propionate, 28, 29
Halog, 29
Heart disorders, exercise and, 96
Herbs
    about, 83
    types of, 83–85
Histamines, 19
Hormones, psoriasis and, 16–19
Hydrea, 36

Hydrochloric acid, 121
    signs and symptoms of low, 122
Hydrocortisone, 30
Hydrocortisone acetate, 30
Hydrocortisone valerate, 30
Hydroxyurea, 36
Hypoglycemia, 18

I
Ibuprofen. *See* Nonsteroidal anti-inflammatory drugs.
IL-2 fusion toxin, 41
Immune system health, foods and, 120–121, 123–124
Immune therapy, 40–41
Infection, psoriasis and bacterial, 22
Inflammation, foods that help reduce, 119–120
Ingram regime, the, 33
Insomnia, 98
Insulin, 17
Inverse psoriasis, 10
Iron-rich foods, 118
Isotretinoin, 38, 40

K
Kenalog, 29
Koebner phenomenon, 7

L
Lasan, 32
Laughter, power of, 110
Lecithin, 88–89
Lidex, 29

Panax ginseng. See Ginseng.

Pancreas, 17–18

Pantothenic acid. *See* Vitamin
   B$_5$.

Pauling, Dr. Linus, 77

PGE1. *See* Prostaglandin E1.

Phosphorus-rich foods, 118

Phototherapy, 32–34

Plaque psoriasis, 9–10

Polyamines, 21, 22, 86

Posture, maintaining good,
   101

Potassium-rich foods, 118

Prograf, 41

Prostaglandin E1 (PGE1), 25

Prostaglandins, 23, 24, 119

Psoralen, 33, 34

Psorcon, 28, 29

Psoriasis
   about, 6–7
   allergies and, 19–20
   causes of, 8–9, 15–26
   controlling, guidelines for,
      44–45
   diet for repelling, 99–100.
      See also Anti-psoriasis diet.
   essential fatty acid
      deficiencies and, 23–25
   free radicals and, 22
   healthy habits for
      controlling, 94–110
   hormones and, 16–19
   identifying causes of, 46–55
   lifestyle changes for
      treating, 56–58, 94

medical attitude towards
   natural treatments for,
   58–62

nutritional supplements for,
   55, 63–65, 65–89

other skin disorders and, 12

stress and, 16, 131–132

symptoms of, 8

topical treatments for, 28–32

toxic substances and, 21–22

treatments for, common,
   11–12, 27–42

types of, 9–11

vitamin and mineral
   deficiencies and, 22–23

who is affected by, 9

Psoriasis Cure Program, 43–62
   guidelines for following,
      44–45
   steps for following, 46–47,
      54–62

Psoriasis vulgaris, 9

Psoriatic arthritis, 7–8

Pustular psoriasis, 10

PUVA therapy, 33–34

Pyridoxine. *See* Vitamin B$_6$.

R

Rapid eye movement (REM)
   sleep, 97–98

Relationships, managing, 137

Relaxation techniques,
   133–135

REM sleep. *See* Rapid eye
   movement (REM) sleep.

Resistance, the body's
   response to, 131